BORDERLINE PERSONALITY DISORDER IN OLDER ADULTS

EMPHASIS ON CARE IN INSTITUTIONAL SETTINGS

Whether at age 30 or 75, anyone who stops learning is old; but anyone who keeps learning stays young. Explore this book, question it and turn it inside out!

with appreciation,

Ana Hategan
Nov 25, 2015 ☺

PSYCHIATRY - THEORY, APPLICATIONS AND TREATMENTS

Additional books in this series can be found on Nova's website under the Series tab.

Additional e-books in this series can be found on Nova's website under the e-book tab.

BORDERLINE PERSONALITY DISORDER IN OLDER ADULTS

EMPHASIS ON CARE IN INSTITUTIONAL SETTINGS

ANA HATEGAN, MD
JAMES A. BOURGEOIS, OD, MD
GLEN L. XIONG, MD, CMD
EDITORS

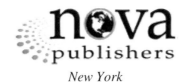

nova publishers

New York

NOTICE TO THE READER

Library of Congress Cataloging-in-Publication Data

ISBN: 978-1-63482-221-3
Library of Congress Control Number: 2015932301

Published by Nova Science Publishers, Inc. † *New York*

*This book is dedicated to our colleagues of many professional disciplines
caring for older adults in various clinical settings,
to the patients whom we hope to help through more understanding, and
to Drs. Marie-France Tourigny-Rivard, Jerald Kay, Molly Hall,
and Wei Jiang,
tireless mentors who shaped us, taught us, and inspired us.*

CONTENTS

FOREWORD

Calvin Hirsch, MD

Professor of Clinical Internal Medicine (Geriatrics) and Public Health Sciences
University of California, Davis Health System,
Sacramento, CA US

Although borderline personality disorder (BPD) has a prevalence of ~ 6% in the primary care setting, the condition easily can be misdiagnosed or missed altogether by non-psychiatrists in older patients. Debilitating symptoms associated with BPD can be ameliorated with a combination of psychotherapy and pharmacotherapy, although data for the efficacy of individual drugs are based on small clinical trials and observational studies. Failure to recognize BPD and to collaboratively develop effective interventions not only may prevent gains in quality of life, but may subject vulnerable patients to inappropriate, potentially harmful treatments and deprive family and institutional caregivers of the tools they need to effectively care for the patient, as well as to handle the negative transference that commonly occurs.

BARRIERS TO RECOGNITION

The hazards of specialty-driven "illness scripts": The constellation of affective dysregulation, anger outburts, black-and-white thinking, poor decision-making, self-neglect, failure to thrive, and strained interpersonal relationships can be attributed to conditions other than BPD that are more commonly seen in older patients, such as dementia, isolated depression, multi-organ chronic illness, and elder mistreatment. Primary care providers are trained to take an organ-system approach to acute and chronic illness and may not explore psychosocial issues unless raised by the patient. Constrained by short visit times, they rely on "illness scripts," which are patterns of clinical presentation that trigger specific differential diagnoses and set priorities for diagnostic and therapeutic interventions. Although geriatrics emphasizes the incorporation of functional and psychosocial issues into clinical decision-making, geriatricians, too, rely on their own set of "illness scripts" as a shortcut to diagnosis and management. If an older patient appears not to be taking her medications, is losing weight, and making frequent visits to the emergency department, concern for self-neglect would be raised. In the Chicago Health and Aging Project, the prevalence of self-neglect in persons aged 65+ had a prevalence of 2.4% in whites and 13.2% in blacks, was present in

14.7% of seniors with less than a high-school education, and was found in 21.7% of seniors with an annual income of < 15,000 U.S. dollars. [1] Our illness scripts for self-neglect might prompt an assessment for depression or cognitive impairment, but likely would not include BPD unless the patient already carried the diagnosis. If a functionally dependent older adult with BPD claims that her children refuse to help her, the "illness script" of elder abuse might surface, prompting a referral to an adult protective services agency that could further strain relationships within the family and potentially damage the family's therapeutic alliance with the doctor. The patient's BPD as the root cause of the strained relations might go unrecognized.

Time spent on mental-health concerns in primary care: In observed encounters with older patients, primary-care physicians in a variety of practice settings discussed mental-health topics 22% of the time, but only spent an average of 2 minutes per encounter on the mental-health issues. [2] Given the short amount of time devoted to behavioral health in primary care, the rate of prescription of psychotropic medications is disproportionately high. The Third National Health and Nutrition Examination Survey (1988-1994) revealed that 9.9% of patients age 60+ received one or more prescriptions for a psychotropic medication, most often for an anxiolytic, sedative, or hypnotic. [3] These data suggest that, as a group, primary-care physicians readily treat symptoms associated with behavioral health disorders, but may be missing or misdiagnosing complex behavioral disorders like BPD.

Barriers in long-term care: Recognition of BPD in skilled nursing facilities is hampered by poor training of staff and the often-superficial nature of the mandated monthly visits by physicians and nurse practitioners/physician assistants. Required training for nursing assistants in assisted living facilities is even less. Staff complaints of "agitated behavior," often poorly characterized, frequently are accompanied by requests for tranquilizers. For behavioral disturbances, missing information about the frequency and severity, associated factors, effective and ineffective management strategies, and patterns of interaction with staff hamper correct diagnosis and proper management. It is unknown how often institutionalized patients who have angry outbursts and "agitated" behavior related to BPD are lumped in with all other patients with disruptive behavior. A lack of accessible and accurate information about patients is considered a severe problem in nursing homes, based on the average rating by respondents to a survey of medical directors. [4] Antipsychotic drugs are prescribed to about a third of patients in U.S. nursing homes who are diagnosed with dementia. Facilities with higher use of antipsychotics tend to be larger, urban, and understaffed. [5, 6] In a study of facilities with access to psychiatric consultation, the use of antipsychotics varied two-fold among consultant groups (range 12.2% to 26.4%), even after adjusting for resident case-mix and facility characteristics. [7] To the geriatrician or primary-care physician, this variation in practice patterns should be unsettling. Some of the variation could be explained by differences in the quality of patient information made available by the facility and the family to the consulting psychiatry group.

Access to mental health services for older patients in the U.S.: In the 2004-2005 Community Tracking Study, 66.8% of non-federal primary-care physicians surveyed reported that they were unable to obtain high-quality outpatient mental-health services for their patients, compared to 33.8% for inability to obtain high-quality specialist referrals. [8] Starting in January, 2014, Medicare required 100% parity in the percent reimbursed to mental-health professionals of allowed charges, compared to the percent reimbursed to other specialists. However, the formulae for reimbursement heavily weight the higher overhead of proceduralists compared to the cognitive specialties, resulting in overall lower reimbursement rates for psychiatrists and psychologists. Medicare's payments to clinical psychologists declined a cumulative 24% between 2007 and 2013, [9] creating a disincentive to provide psychotherapy to Medicare recipients outside of managed care plans. Psychotherapy, an important element in the treatment of BDP in the older patient, may be difficult to obtain in some communities.

Fragmentation and the loss of continuity of care: In the present U.S. health-care system, care is fragmented between the hospital, outpatient clinic, emergency department, and the nursing home, especially in metropolitan areas. Outpatient specialty care adds to the fragmentation, with treatment often initiated and modified by specialists instead of recommended to the primary-care provider, the traditional coordinator of care. Acute-care clinicians tend to focus on the acute illness and may miss clues to an underlying BPD unless there is documentation in the patient's institutional medical record, which often does not include mental health records.

A 61-year-old man is admitted to the orthopedic service from a nursing home after standing up from his wheelchair and losing consciousness, sustaining a right shoulder fracture. He has a history of type 1 diabetes mellitus that has been poorly controlled due to medication non-adherence. Complications include severe autonomic neuropathy with profound orthostatic hypotension, despite severe supine hypertension. As an inpatient, he intermittently refuses his insulin despite blood sugars over 400 mg/dl, refuses to wear compression stockings despite several pre-syncopal episodes from orthostatic hypotension, walks to the bathroom alone against physician orders, and routinely becomes hostile to and "fires" some of his doctors and nurses, while remaining polite to others. At the nursing facility he had been placed on olanzapine because of frequent agitation and angry outbursts, and carried a diagnosis of schizoaffective disorder. Family reported that he abused marijuana and alcohol at the facility. A psychiatric consultation is called in the hospital to assess him for BPD. He is somewhat hostile to the consulting psychiatrist and declines to discuss his background or current psychosocial situation. The psychiatrist finds him to have limited judgment and insight, concrete thinking, no delusional beliefs, and no evidence of homicidal or suicidal ideation, but considers him to be mildly depressed. The psychiatrist is concerned about delirium and a substance-abuse disorder, and recommends low-dose olanzapine and follow-up with the psychiatric consultant to the nursing home "who knows him better." No diagnosis of BPD is made.

The acute-care setting, in which the older patient may be very ill, delirious, or under the influence of opiates, anticholinergics, or other medications that could affect cognition, can be a poor environment in which to evaluate a patient for BPD. In primary care it is not uncommon for patients to be pinned with an inaccurate diagnosis ("chart lore") that sticks with them and which treating physicians accept as truth, thereby perpetuating the misdiagnosis and hampering re-analysis of the symptoms. It is likely that the same applies to complex psychiatric disorders like BPD. In the modern era, these patients transition from one primary-care provider to another, from one health system to another, and from one acute-care setting to another. In a fragmented healthcare environment, the continuity of care that allows symptoms that arise over time to be connected into a pattern fitting the diagnosis of BPD may never occur. As in this patient, certain behavioral disorders may emerge that label the patient as having one or more psychiatric illnesses, but the dots revealing the classic signs and symptoms of BPD never are connected.

As this book reveals, recognition of BPD in older patients may be particularly challenging. It is a diagnosis to which primary-care physicians, hospitalists, and emergency-room physicians – not just psychiatrists – need to be attuned. For general internists and family physicians interested in mental health issues (and all should be), this book provides valuable information about clues to making the diagnosis and insight into its optimal management in the older patient. Even though the length of continuity of care today may be measured in years, rather than decades, primary-care physicians have the greatest opportunity to pick up valuable clues that would place BPD on their list of differential diagnoses, if they were educated about its presentation. Providing the psychiatrist with these clues, gathered over months to years of longitudinal follow-up, could facilitate making a formal diagnosis and instituting appropriate therapy.

Psychotropic medication has the potential for serious complications in older patients, ranging from an increased risk of all-cause mortality with antipsychotics to an increased risk of falls with serotonin agonists and gait instability from anticonvulsant mood stabilizers. The types and doses of psychotropic medication should be determined based on a close collaboration with primary-care providers and shared medical records, rather than selected and started in isolation. Integrated psychiatric and primary care may increase the number of primary-care visits but reduces costly visits to the ED, [10] and represents a model for the management of BPD. Those who furnish medical care to older patients and confront their mental as well as physical illnesses will find this book informative and a valuable reference.

REFERENCES

[1]   Dong X, Simon MA, Evans DA. Prevalence of self-neglect across gender, race, and socioeconomic status: findings from the Chicago Health and Aging Project. *Gerontology*. 2012; 58(3):258-268.

[2]   Tai-Seale M, McGuire T, Colenda C, Rosen D, Cook MA. Two-minute mental health care for elderly patients: inside primary care visits. *J Am Geriatr Soc*. 2007; 55(12): 1903-1911.

[3]   Paulose-Ram R, Jonas BS, Orwig D, Safran MA. Prescription psychotropic medication use among the U.S. adult population: results from the third National Health and Nutrition Examination Survey, 1988-1994. *J Clin Epidemiol*. 2004; 57(3): 309-317.

[4]   Caprio TV, Karuza J, Katz PR. Profile of physicians in the nursing home: time perception and barriers to optimal medical practice. *J Am Med Dir Assoc*. 2009; 10(2): 93-97.

[5]   Kamble P, Chen H, Sherer JT, Aparasu RR. Use of antipsychotics among elderly nursing home residents with dementia in the US: an analysis of National Survey Data. *Drugs Aging*. 2009; 26(6): 483-492.

[6]   Kleijer BC, van Marum RJ, Frijters DH, Jansen PA, Ribbe MW, Egberts AC, et al. Variability between nursing homes in prevalence of antipsychotic use in patients with dementia. *Int Psychogeriatr*. 2014; 26(3): 363-371.

[7] Tjia J, Field T, Lemay C, Mazor K, Pandolfi M, Spenard A, et al. Antipsychotic use in nursing homes varies by psychiatric consultant. *Med Care.* 2014; 52(3): 267-271.

[8] Cunningham PJ. Beyond parity: primary care physicians' perspectives on access to mental health care. *Health Aff (Millwood).* 2009; 28(3): w490-501.

[9] Communications Staff. What's the Problem with Medicare Payment? Practice Update: American Psychological Association, Aug. 29, 2013. http://www.apapracticecentral.org /update/2013/08-29/medicare-payment.aspx. Accessed February 15, 2015.

[10] Druss BG, Rohrbaugh RM, Levinson CM, Rosenheck RA. Integrated medical care for patients with serious psychiatric illness: a randomized trial. *Arch Gen Psychiatry.* 2001; 58(9): 861-868.

PREFACE

On clinical rounds at an academic medical center, a clerkship medical student concisely and poignantly (if inadvertently) summarized a common clinical experience when he began his case presentation: "The patient is a 66-year-old white female who was admitted from the emergency department with an exasperation (sic) of borderline personality disorder." The painful life experiences of borderline personality disorder patients often include long period of self-doubt/self-loathing, interpersonal turbulence, self-destructive behavior, and great difficulties in tolerating and maintaining interpersonal intimacy. Due to their borderline personality disorder, multiple psychiatric comorbid illnesses, substance use disorders, and often, chronic systemic illnesses, these patients are high utilizers of psychiatric and systemic medical care. Because of their difficulties with coping with distress, poor frustration tolerance, and tendency to crisis presentations, they are known to create behavior problems in medical settings. Not surprisingly, they evoke much negative countertransference in health professionals, some of whom actively avoid dealing with them. The patients often engage in a pas-de-deux of "hostile dependency" on care delivery systems, wherein they demand high intensity treatment, only to then sabotage the efforts of others to help them. Understandably, but regrettably, medical personnel react to this with negative responses and use of discriminatory and prejudicial language reflecting these challenges.

In recent years, there has been an increasing progress on the clinical phenomenology, diagnostic clarity, appreciation of psychiatric comorbidity, and the development of better clinical interventions for borderline personality disorder. That *is* to the good, as a common descriptive language, clarity of understanding of clinical phenomena, and application of evidence-based interventions has led to an era of greater empathic understanding treatment approaches that are more than therapeutic nihilism--all resulting in better outcomes. Nevertheless, further work is to be done on borderline personality disorder, especially in older adults. This diagnosis is often forgotten or overlooked within geriatric care delivery systems despite research and clinical experience showing that the core features of borderline personality disorder (albeit with its intrinsic age-related clinical transmutation) continue to be disabling. Facilitating adaptation of service provision to better meet the needs of older patients with borderline personality disorder remains an imperative.

The editors were motivated to mobilize our many chapter authors to compose this book based on years of experience in medical center-based psychosomatic medicine (JAB), geriatric psychiatry (AH), and inpatient psychiatry and long-term care facilities (GX). There is already a well-established literature on borderline personality disorder in the general hospital setting. Yet, as the population ages and becomes chronically "sicker", there is a need for understanding the experience of patients with borderline personality disorder in other care delivery systems, including institutional settings.

Care for patients with borderline personality disorder can be challenging. These patients are prone to emotional dysregulation, crisis presentation, negotiations with medical and nursing staff, and splitting. In the current era of shortened hospital stays, there is a need for guidance in the management of borderline personality disorder in health care settings other than the general hospital. In many settings, such as rehabilitation units and nursing homes, length of stay is much longer than in the general hospital and there is thus more opportunity for patients with behavioral problems to engage in problematic relationships with staff members. Common challenges such as dealing with medical illness and impending mortality, which are difficult for most patients, are magnified in patients with poor coping skills and dysfunctional distress tolerance at baseline.

We hope that this book is useful to many groups of clinicians. For psychiatrists and allied mental health professionals, this book serves as a concise review of borderline personality disorder, psychiatric comorbidity, and psychiatric and social interventions. For other physicians, nurses, and other health professionals, this is an update of the current thinking and a more hopeful approach to clinical management from a stance of greater understanding. Most importantly, we hope to articulate a clear language of understanding, both for patients to feel understood, and for clinicians to understand these patients better. From that stance of greater mutual understanding and validation, clinical interventions may be more successful. For health care administrators, this book can explain the experience of these patients in institutional settings, so as to provide for adequately informed and integrated systemic medical and psychiatric care resources that align in an integrated, rather than fragmented, care model. Indeed, the integrated care and management approach to borderline personality disorder may be directly applicable to other institutionalized patients as well.

Finally, for the patients who experience borderline personality disorder, often among the most disabling of all psychiatric illnesses, we hope that describing their inner worlds in a way that enhances empathic understanding, there may be opportunities for more patient-centered care in institutional settings that minimizes suffering and optimizes opportunities for better clinical outcomes. We hope that this results in better care experiences as they confront the challenges of aging, infirmity, and mortality.

Ana Hategan, MD
James A. Bourgeois, OD, MD
Glen L. Xiong, MD, CMD

CONTRIBUTORS

Mariam Abdurrahman, MD, MSc, FRCPC McMaster University, Hamilton, ON, Canada

Yuri A. Alatishe, MD, FRCPC
Assistant Clinical Professor of Psychiatry and Forensic Psychiatrist,
St. Joseph's Healthcare Hamilton,
Department of Psychiatry and
Behavioural Neurosciences,
McMaster University,
Hamilton, ON Canada

Daniel L. Ambrosini, LLB/BCL, MSc, PhD
Assistant Professor and Legal Counsel,
Forensic Psychiatry Program,
St. Joseph's Healthcare Hamilton,
Department of Psychiatry and
Behavioural Neurosciences,
McMaster University,
Hamilton, ON, Canada

Andrew M. Bein, PhD, LCSW
Professor, Division of Social Work,
California State University,
Sacramento, CA, US

Peter Bieling, PhD, CPsych
Clinical Psychologist and Associate
Professor, Department of Psychiatry
and Behavioural Neurosciences,
McMaster University,
St. Joseph's Healthcare Hamilton,
Hamilton, ON, Canada

James A. Bourgeois, OD, MD
Clinical Professor of Psychiatry and
Vice-Chair Clinical Affairs,
Department of Psychiatry/
Langley Porter Psychiatric Institute,
University of California San Francisco,
Consultation-Liaison Service, University
of California San Francisco Medical
Center, San Francisco, CA, US

Caroline Giroux, MD
Assistant Clinical Professor and
APSS Stockton Clinic Medical Director,
Site Director for Clerkship and Residents
at APSS Stockton,
University of California
at Davis, Sacramento, CA, US

Christina B. Gojmerac, PhD, CPsych
Clinical Neuropsychologist and Associate
Professor (PT), Department of Psychiatry
and Behavioural Neurosciences,
McMaster University,
Clinical Neuropsychology Service and
Seniors Mental Health Program,
St. Joseph's Healthcare Hamilton,
West 5th Campus,
Hamilton, ON, Canada

Elise Hall, MD
University of California San Francisco
and SFVAMC Psychosomatic Medicine
Fellow, Department of Psychiatry,
University of California San Francisco,
San Francisco, CA, US

Gary M. Hasey, MD, MSc, FRCPC
Associate Professor of Psychiatry and
Director of the Donald and Lillian Mair
rTMS laboratory and the ECT Program,
St Joseph's Hospital, Faculty of Health
Sciences, Department of Psychiatry
and Behavioural Neurosciences,
School of Biomedical Engineering,
Department of Electrical and Computer
Engineering, McMaster University,
Hamilton, ON, Canada

Ana Hategan, MD, FRCPC
Associate Clinical Professor of Psychiatry
and Geriatric Psychiatrist, Department
of Psychiatry and Behavioural
Neurosciences, Division of Geriatric
Psychiatry, Michael G. DeGroote
School of Medicine, Faculty of Health
Sciences, McMaster University,
Hamilton, ON, Canada

Calvin Hirsch, MD, FACP
Professor of Clinical Internal Medicine
(Geriatrics) and Public Health Sciences
University of California, Davis Health
System, Sacramento, CA, US

Brian Holoyda, MD, MPH
Psychiatry Resident, University of
California, Davis Medical Center,
Sacramento, CA, US

Julie Hylton, MD
Psychiatry Resident, University of
California, at Davis, Department of
Psychiatry and Behavioral Sciences,
Sacramento, CA, US

Laura Kenkel, MD
Associate Physician Diplomate, Health
Sciences Assistant Clinical Professor,
University of California, at Davis,
Department of Psychiatry and Behavioral
Sciences, Sacramento, California, US

Jelena P. King, PhD, CPsych
Clinical Psychologist and Associate
Professor (PT), Department of
Psychiatry and Behavioural
Neurosciences, McMaster University,
Clinical Neuropsychology Service and
Schizophrenia & Community Integration
Service, St. Joseph's Healthcare Hamilton,
West 5th Campus, Hamilton, ON, Canada

Barbara J. Kocsis, MD
Psychiatry Resident, Department of
Psychiatry and Behavioral Sciences,
University of California, at Davis, School
of Medicine, Sacramento, CA, US

Sheila Lahijani, MD
Psychosomatics Fellow, Northwestern
University Feinberg School of Medicine,
Department of Psychiatry and Behavioral
Sciences, Chicago, IL, US

Margaret W. Leung, MD, MPH
Palliative Medicine Fellow, Harvard
Medical School, Palliative Medicine,
Boston, MA, US

Margaret McKinnon, PhD, CPsych
Clinical Psychologist, Associate Professor
and Associate Chair of Research,
Department of Psychiatry and Behavioural
Neurosciences, McMaster University,
St. Joseph's Healthcare Hamilton,
Homewood Research Institute,
Hamilton, ON, Canada

Heather E. McNeely, PhD, CPsych
Clinical Psychologist and Assistant
Professor, Department of Psychiatry and
Behavioural Neurosciences, McMaster
University, Clinical Neuropsychology
Service and Schizophrenia &
Community Integration Service,
St. Joseph's Healthcare Hamilton,
West 5th Campus, Hamilton, ON, Canada

Liesel-Ann Meusel, PhD
Rotman Research Institute, Baycrest,
Toronto, ON, Canada

Tua-Elisabeth Mulligan, MD
Psychiatry Resident, Department of
Psychiatry, University of California
San Francisco, San Francisco, CA, US

Usha Parthasarathi, MBBS, FRCPC
Associate Clinical Professor of Psychiatry,
Division of Forensic Psychiatry,
McMaster University,
Hamilton, ON, Canada

Karen Saperson, MBChB, FRCPC
Associate Professor of Psychiatry
and Associate Chair of Education,
Department of Psychiatry and
Behavioural Neurosciences, Academic
Head of Division of Geriatric Psychiatry,
Michael G. DeGroote School of Medicine,
Faculty of Health Sciences,
McMaster University,
Hamilton, ON, Canada

Lorin M. Scher, MD
Health Sciences Assistant Clinical
Professor and Director, Emergency
Psychiatry, Psychosomatic Medicine
Service, Department of Psychiatry
& Behavioral Sciences, University
of California, at Davis, School
of Medicine, Sacramento, CA, US

Andreea L. Seritan, MD
Associate Professor of Clinical Psychiatry,
University of California, at Davis,
Department of Psychiatry and Behavioral
Sciences, Sacramento, CA, US

Sid Stacey, MHSc, FCCHL, FACHE
Fellow of the Canadian College of
Health Leaders, Fellow of the American
College of Healthcare Executives,
Director of Administration and
Assistant Professor (PT), Department
of Psychiatry and Behavioural
Neurosciences, Faculty of Health
Sciences, McMaster University,
Hamilton, ON, Canada

Christine Stanzlik-Elliott, MSW, RSW
Discharge Specialist,
St. Joseph's Healthcare Hamilton,
West 5th Campus, Hamilton, ON, Canada

Shannon Suo, MD
Associate Clinical Professor, University
of California, at Davis, Department of
Psychiatry and Behavioral Sciences,
Sacramento, CA, US

Albina Veltman, MD, FRCPC
Associate Professor of Psychiatry,
Department of Psychiatry and Behavioural
Neurosciences, Diversity & Engagement
Chair, Undergraduate MD Program,
Michael G. DeGroote School of Medicine,
Faculty of Health Sciences,
McMaster University,
Hamilton, ON, Canada

Jessica E. Waserman, MD
Psychiatry Resident, Department
of Psychiatry and Behavioural
Neurosciences, Michael G. DeGroote
School of Medicine, Faculty of Health
Sciences, McMaster University,
Hamilton, ON, Canada

Tricia K.W. Woo, MD, MSc, FRCPC
Associate Professor, Division of
Geriatric Medicine, Department
of Medicine, McMaster University,
Hamilton, ON, Canada

Glen L. Xiong, MD, CMD
Health Sciences Associate Clinical
Professor of Psychiatry, Department of
Psychiatry and Behavioral Sciences,
University of California, at Davis,
Sacramento, CA, US

COVER ILLUSTRATION BY:
Caroline Giroux, MD

SECTION I

FUNDAMENTALS OF BORDERLINE PERSONALITY DISORDER IN OLDER ADULTS

In: Borderline Personality Disorder in Older Adults
Editors: A. Hategan, J. A. Bourgeois, G. L. Xiong

ISBN: 978-1-63482-221-3
© 2015 Nova Science Publishers, Inc.

Chapter 1

OVERVIEW OF BORDERLINE PERSONALITY DISORDER IN OLDER PATIENTS: EVOLUTION AND COMPLEXITY

James A. Bourgeois[1,], OD, MD, Ana Hategan[2], MD,*
Albina Veltman[3], MD, and Elise Hall[4], MD

[1]Clinical Professor, Psychiatry, Department of Psychiatry/Langley Porter
Psychiatric Institute, University of California San Francisco, CA, US
Consultation-Liaison Service, University of California San Francisco
Medical Center, San Francisco, CA, US
[2]Associate Clinical Professor, Psychiatry Department of Psychiatry
and Behavioural Neurosciences, Michael G. DeGroote School of Medicine,
Faculty of Health Sciences, McMaster University, Hamilton, ON, Canada
[3]Associate Professor of Psychiatry, Department of Psychiatry
and Behavioural Neurosciences and Diversity & Engagement Chair,
Undergraduate MD Program, Michael G. DeGroote School of Medicine,
Faculty of Health Sciences, McMaster University,
Hamilton, ON, Canada
[4]University of California San Francisco and SFVAMC Psychosomatic
Medicine Fellow, Department of Psychiatry, University of
California San Francisco, San Francisco, CA, US

Borderline personality disorder (herein referred to as BPD) is commonly a lifelong affliction, associated with high utilization of psychiatric and non-psychiatric health services, usually initially manifest by young adulthood and persistent throughout the lifespan. However, clinical recovery is possible for many BPD patients with appropriate psychiatric care. Many others, however, especially those patients with poor treatment engagement, continue to suffer various psychiatric morbidities throughout life. The specific symptoms and behaviors can change over time and understanding of the evolution of this disorder and its clinical manifestations over time are important in order

* Corresponding author: james.bourgeois@ucsf.edu

to properly identify, treat, and serve these patients. The clinical diagnostic criteria for BPD have also evolved over time, but specific considerations of BPD in older adults have yet received little attention in the medical literature. This chapter illustrates the general principles of BPD, history of the diagnosis, and the clinical characteristics and associated risks for disruptive life events in older patients with BPD. Although descriptions in this text primarily pertain to older adults with BPD who are admitted or residing in institutional settings, many of these principles are also applicable to those who are living in the community. Unless otherwise specified, "geriatric" and "older adults" will refer to those aged 65 years or older.

BORDERLINE PERSONALITY DISORDER: GENERAL CONSIDERATIONS

Personality disorders are defined as enduring patterns of inner experience and behavior [1] but the "enduring" aspect may be relative. Some have suggested that personality may show a dynamic course during adulthood, with symptoms more adaptable in early adulthood [2].

In this view, Stone [3] described that the characteristic disturbances of BPD may reemerge in later life following a state of quiescence in mid-adulthood. BPD is an important psychiatric condition to acknowledge because these patients suffer psychiatric instability in several important domains of life based on the personality disorder itself, and experience multiple psychiatric comorbid illnesses.

BPD is one of the psychiatric conditions associated with extensive utilization of psychiatric and non-psychiatric health services (including inpatient, substance use, and emergency services) [4, 5]. The adage that "psychiatric illness is medically expensive" is well illustrated by BPD in many areas. This is true of routine outpatient services (which are relatively low cost), medical emergency services (e.g., for the management of suicide attempts and/or behavioral crisis), and inpatient hospital services (e.g., management of toxic overdoses, trauma services for self-inflicted wounds, and medical complications of substance abuse).

As illustrated later in this book, the psychiatric comorbidities may often be the focus of initial clinical attention (e.g., major depressive, bipolar, anxiety, posttraumatic stress disorder, and substance use disorders). An important association is seen between BPD and intellectual disability (formerly called mental retardation). As such patients may be in need of institutional models of care and placement, consideration of this comorbidity of BPD may be important in their management. Nugent [6] suggests that BPD occurs in people with intellectual disability at rates well above those in the general population.

Some of the characteristics which are reported by staff caring for people with intellectual disability that are associated with BPD include overreacting to typical requests, verbal aggression that is personally disturbing to the victim, over-attachment to some staff and devaluation of others, and extreme changes of mood in disproportionate response to environmental events [7].

Gabriel [8] points out that individuals with intellectual disability and BPD are often volatile and difficult to support. Although there has not been much research published on older patients with developmental disabilities and comorbid BPD, it is obvious from the research on younger patients that caring for these individuals in institutional settings such as group homes poses a significant challenge for staff and therefore, one could easily surmise that the same would hold true for residential facilities caring for older BPD patients.

When patients with BPD attain geriatric age, additional challenges are added. Patients' physical conditions may be compromised in later years by cumulative effects of problematic behavior (e.g., the physical stigmata of prolonged substance abuse, lingering physical limitations from the medical/surgical complications of multiple suicide attempts). Also of interest to medical professionals are the chronic relationship challenges these patients present. Older patients with BPD may have exhausted relationships with well-meaning spouses, children, other relatives, and friends and thus have a very limited network of social support when they are the most in need.

Relationship problems may permeate the physician-patient relationship, in that patients with BPD can be perceived as "dishonest and manipulative," medication-seeking, and non-adherent to medical advice. All of these social and relational problems are magnified when the patient has needs that require ongoing care from others in an institutional setting. Challenges encountered in the management of these patients in specific institutional settings are described in detail in subsequent chapters.

HISTORY OF BORDERLINE PERSONALITY DISORDER: EVOLUTION OF A DIAGNOSIS

The identification of patients as *borderline* first began in the times when psychoanalysis dominated psychiatry [9]. The primary illness category to which these patients were "borderline" was schizophrenia (the patient's behavior "bordered" on psychosis, especially in time of distress) [10]. Kernberg [11] defined *borderline personality organization* as a broad construct of psychopathology lying between neurosis and psychosis and defined by immature defenses such as splitting and projective identification, identity diffusion, and unstable reality testing.

These patients were described as "difficult," "intractable", or "unruly", using institutional settings to evade their responsibilities. They were described with pejorative clinical descriptions that discouraged empathetic understanding [12]. Subsequent efforts were made not only to describe a *borderline syndrome* [13] but also for this syndrome to become reliably diagnosable, with characteristic criteria [14].

By 1980, biological psychiatry had progressed to a place of primacy in psychiatric diagnosis and phenomenology while psychoanalysis began to decline in influence. At that time, the Diagnostic and Statistical Manual of Mental Disorders, third edition (DSM-III) listed BPD as a diagnosable disorder for the first time [15]. The DSM-III inclusion of another new disorder, schizotypal personality disorder (phenomenologically much closer to schizophrenia than was BPD), made it evident that BPD was conceptually unrelated to schizophrenia [16]

It also became evident that ensuing non-psychoanalytic modalities such as the more pragmatic multi-model psychotherapy approaches, including group and family therapy, and pharmacotherapy, could often be helpful for BPD [17].

One of the core symptoms often seen in BPD is identity disturbance. However, the definition of this has evolved over the course of several editions of the DSM. In the DSM-III, identity disturbance was operationalized as an "uncertainty about several issues … such as self-image, gender identity, long-term goals or career choice, friendship patterns, values, and loyalties" [15].

In the subsequent revised edition (DSM-III-R), identity disturbance was defined as "uncertainty about at least two of the following: self-image, sexual orientation, long-term goals or career choice, type of friends desired, or preferred values" [18]. The text in DSM-III referred to "sudden and dramatic shifts" in self-image that included "changes in … sexual identity."

Although the concept of identity disturbance continued to be one of the possible diagnostic criteria for BPD in DSM-IV [19], DSM-IV-TR [20], and now DSM-5 [1], the references to sexual orientation and gender identity have been removed [21]. In the past, transgender individuals were sometimes misdiagnosed as having BPD, but most studies of individuals with gender dysphoria have found no significant comorbidity with BPD on the basis of clinical interviews or standardized psychometric tests [22].

In the 1990s, DSM-IV brought only subtle changes in the definition of BPD. Studies have emerged to show that BPD has a surprisingly good prognosis with treatment [23]. When this was coupled with findings showing a trait heritability of 69% [24], previous theories about BPD's etiology focusing exclusively on environmental causes (e.g., traumatic experiences) started to be contested.

The main differential diagnostic issue had now become bipolar disorder as these conditions are often comorbid and both disorders can demonstrate common diagnostic features pertaining to mood states and can thus overlap phenomenologically [25].

While none of the criteria for personality disorders have changed in the DSM-5, there are some modifications related to coding and classification [1]. Prior to the DSM-5, psychiatric disorders and other health concerns were coded in five separate axes in the DSM. The DSM-5 system combines the first three axes outlined in past editions of the DSM into one axis with all psychiatric and other medical diagnoses. Therefore, BPD and all the other personality disorders no longer falls under Axis II as in DSM-IV because DSM-5 removed the five axial diagnostic convention.

Furthermore, DSM-5 includes an alternative hybrid dimensional-categorical model for personality disorders in which pathological personality traits are considered in conjunction with the degree of impairment in personality functioning. There are 5 broad domains of personality traits, each further subdivided into 25 trait facets. The proposed criteria for BPD include facets from the trait categories of negative affectivity, disinhibition, and antagonism.

Figure 1-1 provides a summary of the evolution of terminology and diagnostic criteria for BPD described previously [1, 11, 13-15, 19].

Despite complicating the course and management of other medical disorders and adversely affecting quality of life, *geriatric* BPD itself has yet to receive significant attention in the literature, nor are there any changes in the diagnostic criteria in older adults within the DSM.

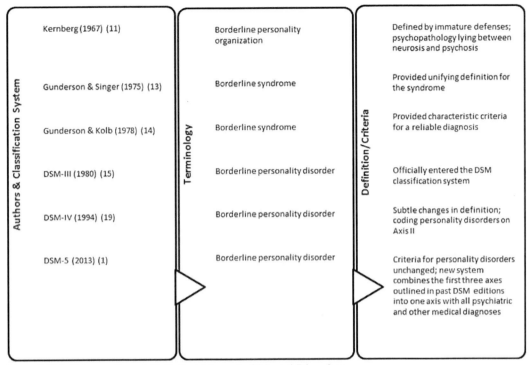

Note: DSM; Diagnostic and Statistical Manual of Mental Disorders.

Figure 1-1. Evolution of Borderline Personality Disorder Terminology and Diagnostic Criteria.

CLINICAL CHARACTERISTICS OF OLDER PATIENTS WITH BORDERLINE PERSONALITY DISORDER

Older patients with BPD are prone to the somatization of distress and may seek medical care for apparent somatic symptoms. The complexity in managing these symptoms may cause difficulties in managing the patient's care within managed care organization and utilization limitations. Such care can result in difficult transferential and countertransferential experiences. The baseline physical frailty of older patients with BPD may make it challenging to see where "real illness" ends and "somatization" begins [26]. These patients' continued stormy interpersonal relations (especially with family members) add further challenge for managing these already complex patients [26].

Of great interest in geriatric psychiatric practice is the assessment and management of mild and major neurocognitive disorders (formerly called dementia). In addition to more clear-cut late-life onset neurocognitive disorders (e.g., Alzheimer's disease) that may be seen in these patients, the presentation of apparent cognitive disorders in older BPD patients may be more subtle and complex, and be associated with the underlying BPD construct. Conversion pseudodementia is a syndrome of apparent cognitive impairment, behavioral regression, and increased interpersonal dependency, which is found (upon full evaluation) not to be due to a clear neurodegenerative dementia syndrome [27]. Due to significant functional impairment, institutional placement is often necessary. In a case series reported by Hepple

[27], he found that a psychiatric history characterized by depression and narcissistic and borderline personality traits was frequent in these patients; he recommended early use of psychotherapy to address the personality disorder component.

A community based longitudinal study of adults ages 55-64 revealed a significant correlation between temperamental and acute BPD symptoms and a history of major depression [28]. Temperamental borderline symptoms (the more enduring, or "trait") remained correlated with major depression, even after correction for the presence of acute BPD symptoms [28].

Patients with BPD reported more emotional distress than patients with other personality disorders [29]. A community sample of 630 middle aged adults, using the Structured Interview for DSM-IV Personality found that BPD was associated with a high level of psychiatric and other mental health treatment-seeking even when corrected for comorbid alcohol dependence and major depression [30]. For older patients with BPD, integration of supportive psychotherapy with active case management may be a useful strategy [31].

Patients with BPD are more likely to experience pain than patients with other personality disorders [32]. They are also more likely to rate their pain as more severe. In a study by Biskin et al. [32], three history items predicted more severe pain complaints among BPD patients: older age, comorbid major depression, and severity of non-sexual childhood abuse. As such, older patients with BPD often may be less responsive to opioid pain medication and may be more prone to unnecessary interventional procedures as the psychological aspects of their pain is less responsive to traditional medical-surgical approaches. Patients with BPD are more prone to opioid dependence. Excess use of benzodiazepines in geriatric patients is a major clinical problem, as these agents are associated with increased risk of falls leading to fractures and cognitive impairment. A study by Petrovic et al. [33] showed a common constellation of symptoms amongst widowed females with BPD that included dysthymic disorder, anxiety disorder, and a predisposition to alcohol dependence, and recommended a psychotherapeutic approach for such older benzodiazepine users. Figure 1-2 presents a summary of these clinical associations with BPD in older adults [26-30, 32, 33].

- Somatization
- Conversion pseudodementia
- Pain
- Major depression
- Anxiety disorder
- Emotional distress
- High level of treatment-seeking
- Excess use of alcohol
- Excess use of opioid pain medications
- Excess use of benzodiazepines

Figure 1-2. Clinical Associations with Borderline Personality Disorder in Older Adults [26-30, 32, 33].

AGE-RELATED DIFFERENCES IN MANIFESTATION OF BORDERLINE PERSONALITY DISORDER

The age-related differences in BPD symptoms are briefly examined here, because a more comprehensive depiction is presented elsewhere in this book. While BPD symptoms often decrease over time, many patients will still meet criteria for BPD in old age [34]. Kenan et al. [35] studied age-related differences in personality disorder diagnosis frequency. Older adults had less frequent personality disorder diagnosis overall, and were specifically less likely to be diagnosed with BPD. These results suggest a decreased experience of BPD in older patients.

In BPD, impulsivity decreases with advanced age, while negative affect persists [34, 36, 37]. A community study in Germany validated the decreased impulsivity with age, whereas depression increased in older adults with BPD compared to younger patients [36]. Similarly, others found that older patients with BPD were less impulsive than younger patients, but continued to experience similar rates of affective disturbance, "identity" disturbance, and interpersonal difficulties [37]. Morgan et al. [34] have shown that, compared to younger patients, older patients with BPD continue to endorse chronic emptiness, have more lifetime hospitalizations, and higher degrees of social impairment, while exhibiting less impulsivity, acts of self-harm, and affective instability.

A mixed clinical and community sample found that older patients with BPD had less impulsivity and fewer suicidal behaviors despite persistent psychological distress [30]. Using a community sample method, De Moor et al. [38] assessed gender and age effects on borderline features. Older women with BPD had less identity problems and affective instability than did the younger women. Figure 1-3 summarizes age-related differences in geriatric patients with BPD compared to the younger counterparts [30, 34, 36-38].

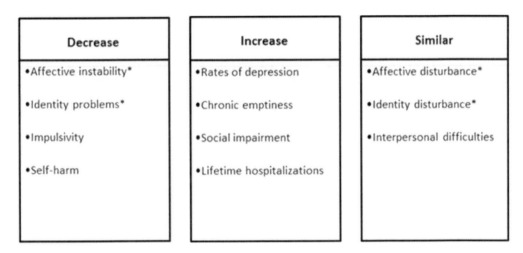

Decrease	Increase	Similar
•Affective instability*	•Rates of depression	•Affective disturbance*
•Identity problems*	•Chronic emptiness	•Identity disturbance*
•Impulsivity	•Social impairment	•Interpersonal difficulties
•Self-harm	•Lifetime hospitalizations	

* Depends on study.

Figure 1-3. Age-Related Differences in Geriatric Compared to Younger Patients with Borderline Personality Disorder [30, 34, 36-38].

RISK FOR DISRUPTIVE LIFE EVENTS IN OLDER PATIENTS WITH BORDERLINE PERSONALITY DISORDER

The older patient with BPD may present for clinical care in the context of disruptive life events; indeed, a crisis presentation in the emergency department or general hospital may be the clinical event that leads to such a diagnostic evaluation and an eventual diagnosis of BPD in the older patient. In a community sample of patients ages 55-64, BPD was associated with an increased frequency of stressful life events [39]. Among the elements of BPD, the areas of unstable interpersonal relationships and impulsivity were associated with increased stressful life events, while feelings of chronic emptiness were associated with a decrease in stressful life events. The latter paradoxical finding may relate to such patients having more social isolation and thus less exposure to interpersonal difficulties.

In a community sample of 1,234 persons ages 55-64, borderline features were also associated with increased frequency of stressful life events even when controlled for concurrent depressed mood [40]. This may be related to affective instability persisting into older age, which predisposes to poorer social functioning. In older adults, posttraumatic stress disorder was most commonly associated with serious illness in the patient or a close contact [41]. In the same population, posttraumatic stress disorder was also associated with BPD and decreased social functioning [41].

In a study of community dwelling older adults, borderline and histrionic personality features were significantly associated with increased suicidal ideation [42]. Suicide rates in older adults correlate to acts of deliberate self-harm. A case control study of self-harming patients found a significant association between a history of personality disorder and acts of self-harm in geriatric patients between ages 65-80 [43]. Among personality traits, borderline and impulsive traits were the most strongly associated with self-harm [43].

KEY POINTS: OVERVIEW OF BORDERLINE PERSONALITY DISORDER IN OLDER PATIENTS: EVOLUTION AND COMPLEXITY

- BPD has long been recognized as common, associated with significant psychiatric comorbidity, and often of long duration across a patient's lifespan.
- The specific symptoms and behaviors can change over time as patients engage various life challenges.
- In geriatric patients with a history of BPD, clinical attention to and understanding of the evolution of the disorder and its clinical manifestations over time are important to properly identify, treat, and serve these patients.
- Older patients with BPD may clinically present in a medical context with suicidal crisis, somatic distress, problematic relationships with medical professionals, prescription medication misuse, and/or neurocognitive disorders.
- The clinical diagnostic criteria for BPD have evolved over time, but relatively fewer studies have been completed on the specific considerations of BPD in older adults. As such, extrapolation of approaches used in other BPD patients (with modifications) may be applied to older BPD patients.

REFERENCES

[1]   American Psychiatric Association. *Diagnostic and Statistical Manual of Mental Disorders*. 5th ed. Arlington, VA: American Psychiatric Publishing; 2013.

[2]   Lenzenweger MF, Johnson MD, Willet JB. Individual growth curve analysis illuminates stability and change in personality disorder features: the longitudinal study of personality disorders. *Arch Gen Psychiatry.* 2004; 61(10): 1015-1024.

[3]   Stone MH. Long-term outcome in personality disorders. *Br J Psychiatry.* 1993; 162: 229-313.

[4]   Bender DS, Dolan RT, Skodol AE, et al. Treatment utilization by patients with personality disorders. *Am J Psychiatry.* 2001; 158(2): 295-302.

[5]   Kvarstein EH, Arnevik E, Halsteinli V, Rø FG, Karterud S, Wilberg T. Health service costs and clinical gains of psychotherapy for personality disorders: a randomized controlled trial of day-hospital-based step-down treatment versus outpatient treatment at a specialist practice. *BMC Psychiatry.* 2013; 13:315. doi: 10.1186/1471-244X-13-315.

[6]   Nugent J. *Handbook on Dual Diagnosis.* Evergreen, CO: Mariah Management; 1997.

[7]   Wilson SR. A four-stage model for management of borderline personality disorder in people with mental retardation. *Mental Health Aspects of Developmental Disabilities.* 2001; 4(2): 68-76.

[8]   Gabriel S. The borderline: Borderline personality disorders in persons with mental retardation. *The National Association for the Dually Diagnosed Newsletter.* 1997; 14(1): 5-9.

[9]   Knight R. Borderline states. *Bull Menninger Clin.* 1953; 17: 1-12.

[10]   Hoch P, Polatin P. Pseudoneurotic forms of schizophrenia. *Psychiatr Q.* 1949; 23: 248-276.

[11]   Kernberg O. Borderline personality organization. *J Am Psychoanal Assoc* 1967; 15: 641-685.

[12]   Houck JH. The intractable female patient. *Am J Psychiatry.* 1972; 129(1): 27-31.

[13]   Gunderson JG, Singer MT. Defining borderline patients: an overview. *Am J Psychiatry.* 1975; 132(1): 1-10.

[14]   Gunderson JG, Kolb JE. Discriminating features of borderline patients. *Am J Psychiatry.* 1978; 135(7): 792-796.

[15]   American Psychiatric Association. *Diagnostic and Statistical Manual of Mental Disorders*. 3rd ed. Washington, DC: American Psychiatric Press, Inc.; 1980.

[16]   Spitzer RL, Endicott J, Gibbon M. Crossing the border into borderline personality and borderline schizophrenia: the development of criteria. *Arch Gen Psychiatry.* 1979; 36(1): 17-24.

[17]   Cloninger CR, Svrakic DM, Przybeck TR. A psychobiological model of temperament and character. *Arch Gen Psychiatry.* 1993; 50(12): 975-990.

[18]   American Psychiatric Association. *Diagnostic and Statistical Manual of Mental Disorders*. 3rd ed. - Revised. Washington, DC: American Psychiatric Press, Inc; 1987.

[19]   American Psychiatric Association. *Diagnostic and Statistical Manual of Mental Disorders*. 4th ed. Washington, DC: American Psychiatric Publishing; 1994.

[20] American Psychiatric Association. *Diagnostic and Statistical Manual of Mental Disorders*. 4th ed. – Text Revision. Washington, DC: American Psychiatric Publishing; 2000.

[21] Singh D, McCain S, Zucker K. Gender Identity & Sexual Orientation in Women with Borderline Personality Disorder. *J Sex Med.* 2011; 8(2): 447-454.

[22] Cole CM, O'Boyle M, Emory LE, Meyer WJ 3rd. Comorbidity of gender dysphoria and other major psychiatric diagnoses. *Arch Sex Behav.* 1997; 26(1): 13-26.

[23] Zanarini MC, Frankenburg FR, Hennen J, Silk KR. The longitudinal course of borderline psychopathology: 6-year prospective follow-up of the phenomenology of borderline personality disorder. *Am J Psychiatry.* 2003; 160(2): 274-283.

[24] Torgersen S, Lygren S, Oien PA, et al. A twin study of personality disorders. *Compr Psychiatry* 2000; 41(6): 416-425.

[25] Belli H, Ural C, Akbudak M. Borderline personality disorder: bipolarity, mood stabilizers and atypical antipsychotics in treatment. *J Clin Med Res.* 2012; 4(5): 301-308.

[26] Trappler B, Backfield J. Clinical characteristics of older psychiatric inpatients with borderline personality disorder. *Psychiatr Q.* 2001; 72(1): 29-40.

[27] Hepple J. Conversion pseudodementia in older people: a descriptive case series. *Int J Geriatr Psychiatry.* 2004; 19(10): 961-967.

[28] Galione JN, Oltmanns TF. The relationship between borderline personality disorder and major depression in later life: acute versus chronic temperamental symptoms. *Am J Geriatr Psychiatry.* 2013; 21(8): 747-756.

[29] Stepp SD, Pilkonis PA. Age-related differences in individual DSM criteria for borderline personality disorder. *J Pers Disord.* 2008; 22(4): 427-432.

[30] Lawton EM, Oltmanns TF. Personality pathology and mental health treatment seeking in a community sample of older adults. *Personal Ment Health.* 2013; 7(3): 203-212.

[31] Clark S. Integration of supportive psychotherapy with case management for older adults with borderline personality disorder. *J Gerontol Soc Work.* 2011; 54(6): 627-638.

[32] Biskin RS, Frankenburg FR, Fitzmaurice GM, Zanarini MC. Pain in patients with borderline personality disorder. *Personal Ment Health.* 2014; 8(3): 218-227.

[33] Petrovic M, Vandierendonck A, Mariman A, van Maele G, Afschrift M, Pevernagie D . Personality traits and socio-epidemiological status of hospitalised elderly benzodiazepine users. *Int J Geriatr Psychiatry.* 2002; 17(8): 733-738.

[34] Morgan TA, Chelminski I, Young D, Dalrymple K, Zimmerman M. Differences between older and younger adults with borderline personality disorder on clinical presentation and impairment. *J Psychiatr Res.* 2013; 47(10): 1507-1513.

[35] Kenan MM, Kendjelic EM, Molinari VA, Williams W, Norris M, Kunik ME. Age-related differences in the frequency of personality disorders among inpatient veterans. *Int J Geriatr Psychiatry.* 2000; 15(9): 831-837.

[36] Arens EA, Stopsack M, Spitzer C, et al. Borderline personality disorder in four different age groups: a cross-sectional study of community residents in Germany. *J Pers Disord.* 2013; 27(2): 196-207.

[37] Stevenson J, Meares R, Comerford A. Diminished impulsivity in older patients with borderline personality disorder. *Am J Psychiatry.* 2003; 160(1): 165-166.

[38] De Moor MH, Distel MA, Trull TJ, Boomsma DI. Assessment of borderline personality features in population samples: is the Personality Assessment Inventory - Borderline

Features scale measurement invariant across sex and age? *Psychol Assess* 2009; 21(1): 125-130.

[39] Powers AD, Gleason ME, Oltmanns TF. Symptoms of borderline personality disorder predict interpersonal (but not independent) stressful life events in a community sample of older adults. *J Abnorm Psychol.* 2013; 122(2): 469-474.

[40] Gleason ME, Powers AD, Oltmanns TF. The enduring impact of borderline personality pathology: risk for threatening life events in later middle-age. *J Abnorm Psychol.* 2012; 121(2): 447-457.

[41] Pietrzak RH, Goldstein RB, Southwick SM, Grant BF. Psychiatric comorbidity of full and partial posttraumatic stress disorder among older adults in the United States: results from wave 2 of the national Epidemiologic Survey on Alcohol and Related Conditions. *Am J Geriatr Psychiatry.* 2012; 20(5): 380-390.

[42] Segal DL, Marty MA, Meyer WJ, Coolidge FL. Personality, suicidal ideation, and reasons for living among older adults. *J Gerontol B Psychol Sci Soc Sci.* 2012; 67(2): 159-166.

[43] Ritchie CW, King MB, Nolan F, et al. The association between borderline personality disorder and an act of deliberate self harm in the older person. *Int Psychogeriatr.* 2011 23(2): 299-307.

In: Borderline Personality Disorder in Older Adults   ISBN: 978-1-63482-221-3
Editors: A. Hategan, J. A. Bourgeois, G. L. Xiong   © 2015 Nova Science Publishers, Inc.

Chapter 2

PERSONALITY AND AGING

Julie Hylton[1,], MD and Andreea L. Seritan[2], MD*

[1]Psychiatry Resident, University of California, Davis
Department of Psychiatry and Behavioral Sciences
Sacramento, CA, US
[2]Associate Professor of Clinical Psychiatry
University of California, Davis
Department of Psychiatry and Behavioral Sciences
Sacramento, CA, US

Typical personality development as well as personality disorders across the life cycle are discussed here, with particular attention to borderline personality disorder (BPD). The five-factor model provides a well-known framework for considering personality. The five domains, including neuroticism, extraversion, openness to experience, agreeableness, and conscientiousness, are briefly examined. BPD has a heterogeneous course with a longitudinal trajectory that will be explored in this chapter. Although BPD has a better prognosis than previously recognized, BPD patients continue to have lower psychosocial functioning than patients with other personality disorders.

INTRODUCTION

Personality has been described as the set of organized and relatively enduring psychological traits and mechanisms that influence an individual's interactions with, and adaptations to, the intrapsychic, physical, and social environments [1]. Personality characteristics result from both constitutional factors and life experiences, particularly those that occurred during childhood [2]. Studies show that personality traits are generally stable and pervasive across situations [3]. Personality disorders are constellations of specific traits, associated with dysfunctional relationships and behavior [2].

---

* Corresponding author: julie.hylton@ucdmc.ucdavis.edu

Life experiences contribute to strengthening and refining individual traits that are adaptive and help build resilience [4, 5]. Based on findings from the seminal longitudinal Harvard Study of Adult Development, Vaillant et al. [4] showed that defense mechanisms usually mature with age, allowing individuals to cope more successfully with life stressors. However, in other instances personality traits become maladaptive and have a deleterious impact on interpersonal relationships. This contributes to increased isolation in older individuals, which in turn may accentuate maladaptive traits and further exacerbate interpersonal conflicts. Personality disorder symptoms often, although not always, improve with psychotherapy.

In this chapter, we discuss the typical personality development across the life cycle, with an emphasis on aging and the trajectory of BPD over time. The core BPD symptoms may impact the relationships with caregivers and health care providers and thus constitute barriers to effective management of older patients in inpatient and other institutional settings.

PERSONALITY DEVELOPMENT ACROSS THE LIFE CYCLE

Several general principles underline the current thinking on typical personality development [6]. The *maturity principle* proposes that individuals become more stable, less prone to negative emotions, and generally more affectionate and friendly with age. The *cumulative continuity principle* highlights the stabilization of personality that occurs with age; in part, this is due to the tendency to commit to and to maintain an identity. Lastly, the *corresponsive principle* states that the most likely effect of life experiences on personality development is to deepen the characteristics that led people to those experiences in the first place [6].

The well-known five-factor model posits a theoretical framework of personality that has gained wide consensus since the 1990s [7]. Much of the contemporary research is based on this model, which outlines five higher-order domains representing general dimensions of personality: neuroticism, extraversion, conscientiousness, openness, and agreeableness [8]. Each of the factors is further divided into six facets, for a total of 30 facets [9]. For illustrating the five-factor model domains, facets, and typical lifetime course, please see Table 2-1 [6, 8, 9]. The five factors will be briefly described below:

- Neuroticism, often described as negative emotionality, can be conceptualized as one's tendency to experience the environment as threatening, endangering, or distressing. Neuroticism may manifest in two ways: inwardly displayed as anxious distress, with tendencies toward sadness, guilt, or insecurity; or more outwardly focused (irritable distress) with tendencies toward anger, hostility, or jealousy [6, 8].
- Extraversion, or positive emotionality, describes one's tendency to actively seek and experience the surrounding world. Central features of extraversion include: sensitivity to potential rewards, the tendency to experience frequent positive moods, and the tendency to enjoy social attention [6].
- Openness to experience is commonly associated with creativity, curiosity, intelligence, and insightfulness [6, 8].

- Agreeableness is a composite of several traits related to maintaining interpersonal harmony: trust, honesty, compliance, interpersonal deference, altruism, and compassion for others [6, 8].
- Conscientiousness, or constraint, speaks to one's degree of control exerted cognitively and in goal-oriented behavior [8]. From a neurobiological standpoint, the degree of conscientiousness may align with attention and executive function [6].

Linear models indicate that conscientiousness and agreeableness increase, while neuroticism, openness to experience, and extraversion tend to decrease with aging [6, 9]. Certain personality phenotypes contribute to poor health decision making, disease onset and progression, and premature mortality [6, 7, 10]. Higher conscientiousness has been shown to be associated with longevity as well as a slower rate of cognitive decline over time [7, 10].

Table 2-1. Factor-Five Model Domains, Facets, and Typical Lifetime Course [6, 8, 9]

Factor Five Domain	Lifetime Course	Facets
Neuroticism	Decrease	Anxiety Depression Hostility Self-consciousness Vulnerability Impulsiveness
Extraversion	Decrease	Excitement-seeking Warmth Gregariousness Energy/activity level Assertiveness Positive emotionality
Openness to experience	Decrease	Values Feelings Actions Fantasy Aesthetics Ideas
Agreeableness	Increase	Trust Straightforwardness Altruism Compliance Modesty Tender-mindedness
Conscientiousness	Increase	Competence Order Dutifulness Achievement striving Self-discipline Deliberation

On the other hand, higher neuroticism, higher extraversion, and lower openness were associated with worse cognitive functioning among 602 older adults (average age at baseline, 79 years) followed prospectively [10]. Costa et al. [11] analyzed longitudinal data from 597 patients aged 66 to 102 and found that straightforwardness (a facet of agreeableness) and self-discipline (an aspect of conscientiousness) were associated with increases in median survival time of 11%, and 34% respectively. Additional facets associated with altruism, imagination, generosity, and higher-quality interpersonal interactions also correlated with increased survival [11]. This echoes the results of the English Longitudinal Study of Ageing, where social isolation and loneliness were associated with worse cognitive function in older adults, perhaps implying that a more agreeable interpersonal style is protective against cognitive decline, by ensuring richer social networks [12]. An increase in emotion-focused, rather than outcome-focused, coping styles also appears to be protective with aging [7].

More recent research indicates that personality traits and well-being reciprocally influence each other over time. In a large sample of Australian residents aged 15 to 93 followed prospectively for five years, higher levels of subjective well-being were associated with higher levels of extraversion, agreeableness, and conscientiousness, and with lower levels of neuroticism [13]. Through a sophisticated analysis using latent growth models and autoregressive models, this study showed that individuals with high initial levels of well-being subsequently became more agreeable, conscientious, emotionally stable, and introverted. Conversely, individuals who were initially more extraverted, agreeable, conscientious, and emotionally stable achieved higher well-being levels over time, reporting higher life satisfaction and positive affect measures [13].

PERSONALITY DISORDERS AND AGING

A growing body of literature has explored the longitudinal trajectories of personality disorder symptoms over time. Unified conclusions are difficult to draw due to:

- age inclusion criteria (adolescents to octogenarians);
- methodological variability (self report, family members' report, or clinician rated instruments);
- setting (inpatient, outpatient, or community dwelling participants);
- availability of and adherence to treatment (pharmacological management, psychotherapy, or both);
- length of follow-up (varying from 2 to 27 years in currently published studies on BPD);
- presence of psychiatric comorbidities;
- presence or absence of a control group [9, 14-21].

Prognosis is impacted by environmental context, genetic vulnerability, and presence of psychiatric comorbidities [3, 21]. A recent study showed that family members reported small, yet significant, increases in personality disorder symptoms over time, despite patients' self-reported improvement [9]. In general, cluster A (i.e., paranoid, schizoid, and schizotypal) and cluster C (i.e., avoidant, dependent, and obsessive compulsive) personality disorder symptoms appear to remain constant or even increase with age, whereas cluster B (i.e., antisocial, borderline, histrionic, and narcissistic) personality disorder symptoms attenuate in late life [2, 15, 20, 22, 23] (Also see Chapter 3).

Gutierrez et al. [20] evaluated patterns of change in personality disorder symptoms in 1,477 patients between ages 15 and 82, by administering a 99-item self-report instrument, the Personality Diagnostic Questionnaire-4+. They found a decline in all personality clusters with age, with the largest reduction in cluster B traits. Specifically, cluster A disorders declined markedly at age 30 and then diverged, with an increase in schizoid personality disorder symptoms and a decrease in schizotypal and paranoid personality disorder symptoms. Cluster B disorders showed a marked decline in the third and fourth decades of life, reaching a low at age 45. Cluster C disorders remained stable until approximately age 35, after which they declined [20].

Case – Mrs. R

Mrs. R was a 71-year-old female with BPD and major depressive disorder, in addition to medical history significant for asthma, congestive heart failure, and osteoarthritis. She had a history of cutting behaviors dating back to her teens, however not in the past thirty years. She had attempted suicide twice, both via overdose. The last attempt occurred in her early 40s, after her second divorce. Mrs. R had three children who all lived within an hour drive of her home, yet she saw each of them only rarely. She had been married twice and had not been in any meaningful relationships since her second divorce. Mrs. R lived alone in a small apartment on a tight income. When she was younger, Mrs. R frequently engaged in spending sprees which she could not afford; these impulsive tendencies lessened over time.

Mrs. R reported a sense of emptiness and loneliness that was fleetingly relieved by isolative hobbies, such as watching cooking shows on TV for hours at a time. Though she denied feeling angry or irritable, her children reported that they experienced her in that way. She felt a desire for social connection, and secretly harbored a fear that her children will not continue to care for her. However, she often rejected their invitations to spend time together at holidays and other family events, becoming anxious and concerned with their perceptions. This hypersensitivity to criticism and rejection often led Mrs. R to assume the worst case scenario, and at times to become suspicious of others' intentions, resulting in further isolation.

BORDERLINE PERSONALITY DISORDER AND AGING

As in the case scenario described previously, BPD is characterized by intense and unstable relationships, affective instability, and impulsive behaviors. BPD has a heterogeneous course over lifetime, with different symptom clusters following different longitudinal patterns [18]. The common externalizing aspects of the disorder – including rule breaking, impulsivity, and emotional turmoil – decrease substantially with age [17]. Impulsive symptoms are most likely to improve over time, including self-mutilating behaviors, suicide attempts, risky sexual behaviors, and substance use [16, 18]. As in Mrs.

R's case, interpersonal impairment continues throughout the lifespan, centered on the BPD patients' insecure attachment patterns [23, 24]. Patients may continue to suffer from dysphoria or other affective symptoms [16]. It is unclear to what degree identity diffusion remains problematic for this population.

Several longitudinal studies have prospectively followed the course of BPD over time, including the Collaborative Longitudinal Personality Study (CLPS) and McLean Study of Adult Development (MSAD) [16-19]. The CLPS was a 10-year study of patients aged 18-45, which compared four personality disorders (avoidant, obsessive-compulsive, borderline, and schizotypal) with one another as well as to MDD in the absence of personality disorders [19]. In this study, 85% of BPD patients remitted, although they had persistent social functioning difficulties [19]. The MSAD followed patients 18-35 years old with BPD as well as other personality disorders for 16 years. Patients with BPD had symptomatic remission rates comparable to other personality disorders [18, 25]. Over the follow-up period, patients with BPD also demonstrated significant improvement on thirteen defense mechanisms, including acting out, emotional hypochondriasis, passive aggression, projection, projective identification, and splitting [18].

In summary, BPD has a better prognosis than previously recognized, with few patients requiring lifelong treatment; however, patients with BPD have been found to have significantly lower psychosocial functioning levels than those with other personality disorders [15, 17-19, 25]. This highlights the critical importance of identifying at-risk individuals, offering early intervention and coordinated management by health care teams, and developing novel therapeutics focused on achieving remission.

KEY POINTS: PERSONALITY AND AGING

- The five-factor model provides a theoretical framework of personality; data suggest that over time, neuroticism, extraversion, and openness decrease, while agreeableness and conscientiousness increase.
- Personality disorder symptoms appear to decrease with age, with the largest decline occurring in cluster B symptoms.
- In BPD, impulsivity symptoms show the largest decreases with age, while affective symptoms often persist.
- BPD has a better prognosis than previously recognized, although many patients continue to suffer functional impairments.

REFERENCES

[1]   Larsen RJ, Buss DM. *Personality psychology: Domains of knowledge about human nature.* 2nd ed. New York: McGraw Hill; 2005:4.

[2]   Abrams RC, Sadavoy J. Personality disorders. In: Sadavoy J, Jarvik LF, Grossberg GT, Meyers BS, eds. *Comprehensive Textbook of Geriatric Psychiatry.* 3rd ed. New York, NY: Norton; 2004: 701-721.

[3]   Hopwood CJ, Morey CL, Donnellan B, et al. Ten-year rank-order stability of personality traits and disorders in a clinical sample. *J Pers.* 2013; 81: 335-344.

[4]   Vaillant GE. The maturing ego. In: *Adaptation to life.* Cambridge, MA: Harvard University Press; 2000: 329-350.

[5]   Boyette LL, van Dam D, Meijer C, et al. Personality compensates for impaired quality of life and social functioning in patients with psychotic disorders who experienced traumatic events. *Schizophr Bull.* 2014; 40: 1356-65.

[6]   Caspi A, Roberts BW, Shiner RL. Personality development: Stability and change. *Annu Rev Psychol.* 2005; 56: 453-484.

[7]   Chapman BP, Robert B, Duberstein P. Personality and longevity: knowns, unknowns, and implications for public health and personalized medicine. *J Aging Res.* vol. 2011, Article ID 759170, 24 pages, 2011. doi:10.4061/2011/759170.

[8]   Costa PT, McCrae RR. *Revised NEO Personality Inventory (NEO–PI–R) and NEO Five-Factor Inventory (NEO–FFI) professional manual.* Odessa, FL: Psychological Assessment Resources; 1992.

[9]   Cooper LD, Balsis S, Oltmanns TF. A longitudinal analysis of personality disorder dimensions and personality traits in a community sample of older adults: perspectives from selves and informants. *J Pers Disord.* 2014; 28: 151-165.

[10] Chapman B, Duberstein P, Tindle HA, et al. Gingko Evaluation of Memory Study Investigators. Personality predicts cognitive function over 7 years in older persons. *Am J Geriatr Psychiatry.* 2012; 20: 612-621.

[11] Costa PT, Weiss A, Duberstein PR, Friedman B, Siegler IC. Personality facets and all-cause mortality among Medicare patients aged 66 to 102 years: A follow-on study of Weiss and Costa (2005). *Psychosom Med.* 2014; 76: 370-378.

[12] Shankar A, Hamer M, McMunn A, Steptoe A. Social isolation and loneliness: relationships with cognitive function during 4 years of follow-up in the English Longitudinal Study of Ageing. *Psychosom Med.* 2013; 75: 161-170.

[13] Soto CJ. Is happiness good for your personality? Concurrent and prospective relations of the Big Five with subjective well-being. *J Pers.* 2013 Dec 3. doi: 10.1111/jopy.12081. [Epub ahead of print].

[14] Stone MH. Long-term outcome in personality disorders. *Br J Psychiatry.* 1993; 162: 299-313.

[15] Paris J, Zweig-Frank H. A 27-year follow up of patients with borderline personality disorder. *Compr Psychiatry.* 2001; 42: 482-487.

[16] Zanarini MC, Frankenberg FR, Hennen J, Silk KR. The longitudinal course of borderline psychopathology: 6-year prospective follow-up of the phenomenology of borderline personality disorder. *Am J Psychiatry.* 2003; 160: 274-283.

[17] Zanarini MC, Frankenberg FR, Hennen J, Reich DB, Silk KR. The McLean Study of Adult Development (MSAD): overview and implications of the first six years of prospective follow up. *J Pers Disord.* 2005; 19: 505-523.

[18] Zanarini MC, Frankenburg FR, Fitzmaurice G. Defense mechanisms reported by patients with borderline personality disorder and axis II comparison subjects over 16 years of prospective follow-up: description and prediction of recovery. *Am J Psychiatry.* 2013; 170: 111-120.

[19]   Gunderson JG, Stout RL, McGlashan TH, et al. Ten year course of borderline personality disorder: psychopathology and function from the Collaborative Longitudinal Personality Disorder studies. *Arch Gen Psychiatry.* 2011; 68: 827-837.

[20]   Gutierrez F, Vall G, Peri JM, et al. Personality disorder features through the life course. *J Pers Disord.* 2012; 26: 763-774.

[21]   Gunderson JG, Stout RL, Shea MT, et al. Interactions of borderline personality disorder and mood disorders over 10 years. *J Clin Psychiatry.* 2014; 75: 829-834.

[22]   Henriques-Calado J, Duarte-Silva ME, Keong AM, Sacoto C, Junqueira D. Personality traits and personality disorders in older women: an explorative study between normal development and psychopathology. *Health Care Women Int.* 2014; 35: 1305-1316.

[23]   Morgan TA, Chelminski I, Young D, Dalyrymple K, Zimmerman M. Differences between older and younger adults with borderline personality disorder on clinical presentation and impairment. *J Psychiatr Res.* 2013; 47: 1507-1513.

[24]   Fossati A, Borroni S, Feeney J, Maffei C. Predicting borderline personality disorder features from personality traits, identity orientation, and attachment styles in Italian nonclinical adults: issues of consistency across age ranges. *J Pers Disord.* 2012; 26: 280-297.

[25]   Gabbard GO. Cluster B personality disorders: Borderline. In: *Psychodynamic Psychiatry in Clinical Practice* .5th ed. Arlington, VA: American Psychiatric Publishing, Inc.; 2014:432-433.

Chapter 3

ETIOLOGY AND EPIDEMIOLOGICAL CORRELATES OF BORDERLINE PERSONALITY DISORDER IN OLDER ADULTS

Mariam Abdurrahman[1],, MD, MSc and Ana Hategan[2], MD*

[1]Psychiatrist, McMaster University, Hamilton, ON, Canada
[2]Associate Clinical Professor of Psychiatry,
Department of Psychiatry and Behavioural Neurosciences,
Division of Geriatric Psychiatry, Michael G. DeGroote School of Medicine,
Faculty of Health Sciences, McMaster University,
Hamilton, ON, Canada

Personality disorders are considered to be life-long and are modulated by interactions between the individual and the environment. However, personality disorders have not been well studied in later stages of life. In the case of borderline personality disorder (BPD), there has been much advance in early to mid-life epidemiology and phenomenology but relatively little is known about BPD in geriatric patients (i.e., aged 65 years and older). A number of retrospective studies have been conducted with the attendant limitations in reliability. More recently, prospective follow-up studies have been conducted but the mean age of participants remains relatively young as they capture patients primarily in early to late middle age. This paucity of research is problematic in that descriptive research and clinical experience show that the core features of BPD continue to be disabling and can be quite disruptive in nursing homes, inpatient geriatric units and other geriatric service delivery settings. This section will summarize the etiology and epidemiological correlates of BPD as it pertains to older adults.

---
* E-mail: mariam.abdurrahman@medportal.ca.

INTRODUCTION

Clinicians evaluating older patients may fail to establish a diagnosis of BPD as the Diagnostic and Statistical Manual, 5th edition (DSM-5) [1] currently does not account for aging related changes in the presentation of personality disorders. Difficulties in establishing a diagnosis of BPD may reflect alterations in the environmental and social context such that core symptoms manifest differently [2]. For example, self-harm may manifest as food refusal while identity disturbance may manifest as an inability to pursue goal-oriented plans. This transmutation is important to recognize within geriatric care delivery systems as it can facilitate adaptation of service provision to better meet the needs of geriatric patients with BPD.

Additional understanding of how geriatric patients with BPD interact with acute and long-term care medical institutions is essential given the worldwide increase in the aging population and the relatively high medical service utilization rates of geriatric patients [3]. Furthermore, the heterogeneity of BPD underscores the need for a more sensitive diagnostic framework to facilitate identification and characterization of BPD, thus allowing for more accurate research and treatment of BPD in an age and phase of life relevant manner.

ETIOLOGY OF BORDERLINE PERSONALITY DISORDER

BPD is a complex multifactorial disorder with a variable phenotype as recognized by the polythetic diagnostic classification systems in use today. The classification of key symptom clusters based on the DSM-5 criteria is shown in Figure 3-1 [1]. Similarly, there is heterogeneity in the etiological factors associated with BPD. The most studied factors include environmental, genetic, neurobiological, and psychological factors [3-6].

Environmental factors: Childhood abuse remains the most consistently and prominently reported environmental factor in BPD [4, 5, 7]. As many as 40-71% of adults with BPD report childhood sexual abuse, while 25-73% report childhood physical abuse in clinical samples of BPD [8].

However, while a notable risk factor and one that discriminates BPD from other personality disorders [9], a history of childhood abuse is not specific to BPD [5]. Rather, adverse early life events such as childhood abuse can produce a variety of pathological sequelae such as BPD in vulnerable populations [5].

- Affective Instability
- Interpersonal Instability
- Identity Instability
- Impulsivity
- Cognitive-perceptive Distortion

Figure 3-1. Key Symptom Clusters based on DSM-5 Criteria for Borderline Personality Disorder [1].

The environmental context may also contribute to seemingly *de novo* cases of BPD in old age, and a resurgence of symptoms in those carrying a previous diagnosis of BPD when critical stressors and growing frailty diminish the capacity to contain internal psychological distress that is imposed by external factors [2]. Furthermore, aging and stage-of-life-related losses may disrupt the "bound borderline personality" through the loss of significant others and significant roles that previously "contained" an individual's character pathology [2]. The manifestation and course of BPD may also be appraised as a mismatch between environment and personality, with some researchers proposing that, over time, individuals with BPD likely select less distressing situations [5], thus performing a form of nidotherapy. This may occur in older patients who minimize interpersonal intimacy and environments that place them in such situations.

Genetic factors: Research is yet to identify any specific genetic risk factors. However, heritability is thought to account for a significant magnitude of the phenomenology of BPD [3]. In a twin study, Torgersen et al. [10] reported a heritability factor of 0.69. However, it is suggested that BPD itself is not inherited as a disorder, but rather it is the traits associated with impulsive aggression and mood dysregulation that are heritable [3]. This is in keeping with an epigenetic mechanism of interplay between adverse environmental experiences and an underlying genetic liability. Core traits, such as affective instability, novelty seeking and impulsivity have been postulated to account for at least half of the variability in most traits studied to date [5, 11].

Neurobiological factors: Neurotransmitter studies have shown associations between BPD and disruption in the central serotonergic system, although specific causal pathways are yet to be identified [3, 4, 11]. BPD has also been associated with disruption in the endogenous opiate pathway, which is implicated in repeated non-suicidal self-harm [3]. A number of studies have examined both anatomical and functional circuitry, and support the hypothesis of dysfunctional frontolimbic networks underlying impulsive aggression and affective dysregulation [3, 4, 11].

Psychological factors: The development of BPD is modulated by a number of predisposing and adverse childhood events in the formative environment (e.g., trauma, neglect) although no conclusive association has been shown between these experiences and the development of psychopathological changes in adulthood [11]. Thus, it is difficult to elucidate the interaction of these factors to any definitive degree.

The etiological factors in BPD discussed previously are summarized in Figure 3-2 [1-7, 10, 11].

EPIDEMIOLOGY OF BORDERLINE PERSONALITY DISORDER IN OLDER ADULTS

Prevalence estimates for personality disorders in the geriatric population are variable, ranging from 2.8-13% in the community, 5-33% among psychiatric outpatients, and 7-61.5% among psychiatric inpatients [12-14]. There are no reliable estimates for BPD. This may be in part due to the fact that most prevalence estimates for personality disorders in the geriatric age group have been extrapolated from chart reviews [13, 14]. Other reasons include difficulties in establishing the diagnosis given the lack of age-adjusted assessment instruments, difficulties of recall bias, and social desirability effects during assessments [15].

Torgersen [16] estimates the median population prevalence of BPD to be 1.6%, but the rate is higher in the National Epidemiological Study on Alcohol and Related Conditions

(NESARC). The second wave of NESARC [17] estimates the lifetime prevalence of BPD at 5.9%, with no significant difference by sex.

In the first wave of the NESARC study [18] only 7 personality disorders were included; BPD was excluded. However, they report that approximately 8% of the geriatric sample of 8,205 individuals presented with at least one personality disorder, with obsessive compulsive personality disorder being the most prevalent.

In Abrams and Horowitz's [19] meta-analysis, the community prevalence of personality disorders in clinical and non-clinical samples at least 50 years of age was estimated at 10%. Moreover, Abrams and Horowitz [19] did not observe a significant difference in the prevalence and cluster of personality disorders between adults above and below the age of 50, despite a widely held impression of lower prevalence of Cluster B (i.e., antisocial, borderline, histrionic, and narcissistic) personality disorders in older adults.

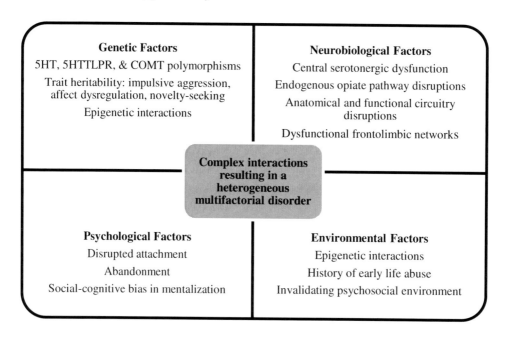

Figure 3-2. Etiological Factors in Borderline Personality Disorder [1-7, 10, 11].

Epidemiological studies of personality disorders have increased significantly over the past decade; however, the number of studies in older adults is relatively limited. Some studies describe a reverse J-shaped distribution for Cluster B disorders, with core traits declining from the fourth to sixth decades of life followed by an upturn and possible resurgence thereafter [2, 13]. Both the International Classification of Diseases and the Diagnostic and Statistical Manual systems of classification conceptualize personality disorders as maladaptive behavioral patterns that appear early (typically by adolescence or early adulthood), are enduring, pervasive, and not limited to episodes of other psychiatric illness.

Given these phenomenological tenets, the limited prevalence data for older adults obscures closer examination of the applicability and stability of these concepts in this age group. In fact, the concept of stability in personality disorders is really more of a case of "stable instability" in the natural history of personality disorders [20]. Relative to the other personality clusters, Cluster B personality disorders have been shown to exhibit the greatest changes over time [20], with the research on BPD increasingly showing a more optimistic outcome than previously thought [21-23]. In fact, BPD has better outcomes than psychiatric disorders such as bipolar and major depressive disorder, where episodic recovery is usually attained more quickly but recurrences are more common [21, 23]. Regardless of age, the data on sex and ethnic distribution of BPD has been equivocal. Some studies report that females account for as many as 80% of those receiving treatment for BPD [6], but community estimates reflect a more balanced sex distribution [3].

Impact of Illness and Functional Correlates: The impact of BPD on social function is evident in the frequent and intense interpersonal crises experienced by affected individuals. In aging patients, the converse may be seen, with increased social withdrawal as a form of self nidotherapy. For individuals engaged in such ego-syntonic isolative behavior in nursing homes, their increasing isolation may raise concerns about clinical depression but they paradoxically fail to respond to treatment. Nonetheless, it is still imperative to evaluate the individual appropriately given the close association between major depression and BPD.

In geriatric patients with comorbid depression, personality disorder symptoms appear to amplify or exacerbate the impact of residual depression on long-term functioning and quality of life [13]. Improvements in BPD are associated with improvements in comorbid depression and functional status. However, the converse is not true; improvement in depressive symptomatology is not accompanied by improvement in borderline personality features.

Lifestyle choices are also affected by BPD symptoms. Relative to unremitted patients with BPD, remitted patients were significantly less likely to report poor lifestyle choices such as smoking, alcohol use, inactivity, and self-medication for sleep and pain in the McLean Study of Adult Development (MSAD) [24].

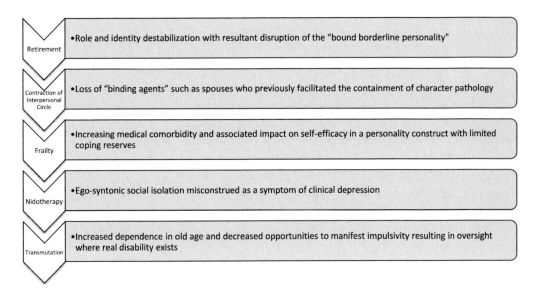

Figure 3-3. Phase of Life Factors in Geriatric Borderline Personality Disorder.

Suicide and other causes of premature death present the most concerning sequelae of BPD. Suicide rates in epidemiological studies range from 4.1% at the 10-year follow up mark in MSAD [24] to 10.3% in Paris and Zweig-Frank's 27-year follow up study [25]. The overall mortality in Paris and Zweig-Frank's Canadian cohort was 18.2%, with 7.9% dying of natural causes between 28 and 56 years of age. The premature mortality associated with BPD is striking, as only 4.5% of Canadian females and 7.5% of males are expected to have died by age 50 [25].

Unfortunately, there is no comparable mortality data for geriatric patients with BPD. Despite the seeming attenuation in clinical presentation with aging, the degree of disability associated with BPD remains significant, making it essential to recognize this disorder in geriatric patients in order to adapt care delivery appropriately. Furthermore, in light of the rapidly growing geriatric population, now is the time for psychiatric researchers to turn their attention to investigating the course of BPD in older adults. Several late-life factors that play a role in BPD and which were discussed above are summarized in Figure 3-3.

KEY POINTS: ETIOLOGY AND EPIDEMIOLOGICAL CORRELATES OF BORDERLINE PERSONALITY DISORDER IN OLDER ADULTS

- There is limited data on the epidemiology of BPD in the latter years of life.
- BPD is a complex disorder of multifactorial etiology, including genetic, neuro-biological, psychosocial, and environmental factors.
- Suicide and premature death present the most concerning sequelae of BPD, however there are currently no reliable estimates for the geriatric age group.
- As the population begins to age more rapidly, now is the time to increase research attention to the phenomenology of BPD in old age.

REFERENCES

[1]   American Psychiatric Association. *Diagnostic and Statistical Manual of Mental Disorders*. 5th ed. Arlington, VA: American Psychiatric Publishing; 2013: 646-649.
[2]   Rosowsky E, Gurian B. Impact of borderline personality disorder in late life on systems of care. *Hosp Community Psychiatry*. 1992; 43(4): 386-389.
[3]   Borderline Personality Disorder: The NICE Guideline on Treatment and Management. National Institute for Health and Care Excellence Web site. http://www.nice.org.uk/ guidance Published January 2009. Accessed June 2, 2014.
[4]   Oldham JM. Guideline Watch: Practice Guideline for the Treatment of Patients with Borderline Personality Disorder. Arlington, VA: American Psychiatric Association. http://www.psych.org/psych_pract/treatg/pg/ prac_guide.cfm. Published March 2005. Accessed May 12, 2014.
[5]   Paris J. Borderline personality disorder. *CMAJ*. 2005; 172(12): 1579-1583.
[6]   Skodol AE, Gunderson JG, Pfohl B, Widiger TA, Livesley WJ, Siever LJ. The borderline diagnosis I: psychopathology, comorbidity, and personality structure. *Biol Psychiatry*. 2002; 51(12): 936-950.
[7]   Zanarini MC, Yong L, Frankenburg FR, et al. Severity of reported childhood sexual abuse and its relationship to severity of borderline psychopathology and psychosocial impairment among borderline inpatients. *J Nerv Ment Dis*. 2002; 190(6): 381–387.

[8]   Zanarini MC. Childhood experiences associated with the development of borderline personality disorder. *Psychiatr Clin North Am.* 2000; 23(1): 89-101.

[9]   Soloff PH, Lynch KG, Kelly TM. Childood abuse as a risk factor for suicidal behavior in borderline personality disorder. *J Pers Disord.* 2002; 16(3): 201-214.

[10] Torgersen S, Lygren S, Øien PA, et al. A twin study of personality disorders. *Compr Psychiatry.* 2000; 41(6): 416-425.

[11] Leichsenring F, Leibing E, Kruse J, New AS, Leweke F. Borderline personality disorder. *Lancet.* 2011; 377(9759): 74-84.

[12] van Alpen SP, Engelen GJ, Kuin Y, Derksen JJ. The relevance of a geriatric sub-classification of personality disorders in the DSM-IV. *Int J Geriatr Psychiatry.* 2006; 21(3): 205-209.

[13] Abrams RC, Bromberg CH. Personality disorders in the elderly. *Psychiatr Ann.* 2007; 37 (2): 123-127.

[14] Ames A, Molinari V. Prevalence of personality disorders in community-living elderly. *J Geriatr Psychiatry Neurol.* 1994; 7(3): 189-194.

[15] Agronin ME, Maletta G. Personality disorders in late life. Understanding and overcoming the gap in research. *Am J Geriatr. Psychiatry.* 2000; 8(1): 4-18.

[16] Torgersen S. The nature (and nurture) of personality disorders. *Scand J Psychol.* 2009; 50(6): 624-632.

[17] Grant BF, Chou SP, Goldstein RB, et al. Prevalence, correlates, disability, and comorbidity of DSM-IV borderline personality disorder: results from the Wave 2 National Epidemiologic Survey on Alcohol and Related Conditions. *J Clin Psychiatry.* 2008; 69(4): 533-545.

[18] Schuster JP, Hoertel N, Le Strat Y, Manetti A, Limosin F. Personality disorders in older adults: findings from the National Epidemiologic Survey on Alcohol and Related Conditions. *Am J Geriatr Psychiatry.* 2013; 21(8): 757-768.

[19] Abrams RC, Horowitz SV. Personality disorders after age 50: a meta-analysis. *J Pers Disord.* 1996; 10(3): 271-281.

[20] Tyrer P, Seivewright H. Stable instability: the natural history of personality disorders. *Psychiatry.* 2008; 7(3): 129-132.

[21] Paris J. The outcome of borderline personality disorder: good for most but not all patients. *Am J Psychiatry.* 2012; 169(5): 445-446.

[22] Skodol AE, Gunderson JG, Shea MT, et al. Collaborative Longitudinal Personality Disorders Study (CLPS): overview and implications. *J Pers Disord.* 2005; 19(5): 487-504.

[23] Zanarini MC. Diagnostic specificity and long-term prospective course of borderline personality disorder. *Psychiatr Ann.* 2012; 42(2): 53-58.

[24] Zanarini MC, Frankenburg FR, Reich DB, Fitzmaurice G. Time to attainment of recovery from borderline personality disorder and stability of recovery: A 10-year prospective follow-up study. *Am J Psychiatry.* 2010; 167(6): 663-667.

[25] Paris J, Zweig-Frank H. A 27 year follow-up of patients with borderline personality disorder. *Compr Psychiatry.* 2001; 42(6): 482-487.

SECTION II

ASSESSMENT AND EVALUATION

In: Borderline Personality Disorder in Older Adults   ISBN: 978-1-63482-221-3
Editors: A. Hategan, J. A. Bourgeois, G. L. Xiong   © 2015 Nova Science Publishers, Inc.

Chapter 4

CLINICAL DIAGNOSIS

Elise Hall[1,], MD and James A. Bourgeois[2], OD, MD*

[1]University of California San Francisco and SFVAMC Psychosomatic Medicine Fellow,
Department of Psychiatry, University of California San Francisco,
San Francisco, CA, US
[2]Clinical Professor, Psychiatry, Department of Psychiatry/Langley Porter Psychiatric
Institute, University of California San Francisco, Consultation-Liaison Service,
University of California San Francisco Medical Center,
San Francisco, CA, US

Borderline personality disorder (BPD) is primarily a clinical diagnosis. It is characterized by a chronic and pervasive pattern of instability in interpersonal relationships, self-image, affects, and marked impulsivity. The categorical classification system for personality disorder assessment of the former Diagnostic and Statistical Manual of Mental Disorders (DSM)-IV system was retained in the present DSM-5 system, in order to maintain continuity with current clinical practice. In this section, we will discuss the diagnostic criteria for BPD, including the alternative, DSM-5 dimensional model for personality disorders. Illustration with case examples and a particular emphasis on application of these diagnostic criteria for geriatric patients with BPD will be endeavored. Some features of BPD, including impulsivity, mature or "burn out" over time, while others, including affective dysregulation, remain resistant to change and stable over time. A brief discussion of clinically practical psychometric instruments, which may be of supplementary value to support the clinical diagnosis, is also included. Barriers to the diagnosis of BPD in geriatric patients are reviewed with a focus on potential resolution of these barriers in order to successfully make this important diagnosis in geriatric patients.

---
[*] Corresponding author: elise.hall@ucsf.edu

DIAGNOSIS

As defined in DSM-IV-TR and DSM-5, BPD is characterized by a chronic and pervasive pattern of instability in interpersonal relationships, self-image, affects, and marked impulsivity [1, 2]. Please see Figure 4-1 for a complete description of diagnostic criteria, including those consistent with DSM-IV-TR/DSM-5 as well as the DSM-5 alternative model for personality disorders as outlined in Section III, Emerging Measures and Models. The DSM criteria for BPD are not modified to reflect age-related changes and may thus lack face validity in an older adult population. Different criteria within the diagnosis of BPD have variable longitudinal patterns over time (e.g., impulsivity decreases with increasing age). There is a dearth of research focusing primarily on the diagnosis of BPD in the older adult cohort with a growing understanding that this population has many periods of transitions, losses, and health problems that serve as stressors and likely lead to dysfunctional behavioral and affective expressions [3].

There is consensus that some features of BPD do mature, or "burn out", with age (e.g., impulsivity). However, temperamental symptoms such as affect dysregulation, inappropriate and chronic anger, and feelings of emptiness tend to be relatively resistant to change and stable over time, and thus remain as sources of clinical attention in geriatric BPD [4-6]. Affect dysregulation and the resulting interpersonal difficulties continue to be core features of BPD in older adults. Furthermore, the fear of abandonment and loss may be exaggerated compared to what one might expect for an individual at that stage of life [7].

The more acute presenting symptoms of BPD, such as impulsivity and self-harming behaviors, often decrease in intensity as an individual ages [4, 8, 9]. However, in some cases these behaviors do not necessarily "decline" over time but simply "transform" in their manifestations. For example, self-injurious behaviors in the older adult population may manifest as food or hydration refusal, medication non-adherence, and other behaviors that sabotage medical care, as also seen in Case 1 below [10-12]. In physically frail patients, self-injurious behaviors such as food or medication refusal can further complicate the clinical management plan, and become particularly upsetting to the treating clinicians. The manifestation of identity disturbance remains less clear in older patients as pivotal and defining life choices related to sexual relationships, marriage, and career choice become less relevant than in earlier stages of life.

In clinically assessing older adult patients thought to have BPD, it is important for the clinician to be aware that fluctuations between idealizing and devaluing others, or *splitting*, continue to be a prominent feature of the clinical presentation and may be acted out in clinician-patient interactions as seen in the case examples below. The geriatric BPD patient's caregiver and/or treatment team are often the targets of these extremes of overvaluation or devaluation. Individuals with BPD often evoke negative countertransference (i.e., redirection of a clinician's feelings or unresolved conflict toward a patient) in therapeutic relationships [9, 10]. On examination there may be evidence of scars from self-injurious behaviors or skin changes related to a history of alcohol or other substance abuse (e.g., flushing, ulcerations). Geriatric patients with BPD may appear older than their stated age for these reasons. The clinician may also note affective lability on assessment evidenced by rapidly shifting emotions or extreme reactivity. Furthermore, as individuals with personality disorders age and develop cognitive impairment, they can become a more extreme "caricature" or "exaggerated" version of their original personality with persistent maladaptive behavior [13]. It is important for the clinician to be aware of the potential for splitting and also to adopt an empathic and validating stance while maintaining appropriate boundaries as needed. The following case examples illustrate how BPD can manifest in the older adult population in various institutional settings and some of the diagnostic challenges that exist.

DSM-IV-TR Criteria	Alternative DSM-5 Proposed Criteria*
Five of nine criteria must be present:	**A.** *Impairment in two or more of four:*
1. Frantic efforts to avoid abandonment	1. Identity (unstable self-image, chronic feelings of emptiness, self-criticism)
2. Unstable and intense interpersonal relationships (i.e., splitting or alternating between extremes of idealization and devaluation	2. Self-direction (instability related to values, goals, aspirations)
3. Unstable self-image	3. Empathy (interpersonal hypersensitivity and decreased ability to recognize feelings/needs of others)
4. Impulsivity leading to self-damaging behaviors (in at least 2 areas)	4. Intimacy (relationships viewed with extremes of idealization and devaluation, unstable and conflicted relationships)
5. Recurrent suicidal or self-mutilating behavior	**B.** *Four or more of seven pathological traits (at least one is 5, 6, or 7):*
6. Marked reactivity of mood leading to affective instability (e.g., episodic dysphoria or irritability)	1. Emotional lability
7. Feelings of emptiness	2. Anxiousness
8. Disproportionate displays of intense anger	3. Insecurity regarding separation
9. Paranoid ideation or severe dissociative symptoms that are transient and stress related	4. Propensity for depressed mood
	5. Impulsive behavior
	6. Risk taking behavior
	7. Hostility

*Alternative DSM-5 model for personality disorders is found in Section III, Emerging Measures and Models of DSM-5.

Figure 4-1. Diagnostic Criteria for Borderline Personality Disorder, adapted from DSM-IV-TR and DSM-5.

Case 1 – Ms. J

Mrs. J, a 68-year-old divorced female living at a nursing home facility, was admitted to a psychiatric unit for the assessment of behavioral problems. She had a past psychiatric history significant for persistent depressive disorder (dysthymia) and a remote suicide attempt in her 30s when she overdosed on prescription medication. She had a medical history significant for mild neurocognitive disorder, hypertension, atrial fibrillation, fibromyalgia, and chronic lower back pain secondary to a herniated disc. As a result of the chronic back pain, she required the use of a wheelchair and was on long-term opioid medication. She had two adult children and described chaotic relationships with both of them. She was divorced and described her marriage as tumultuous and full of conflict. She had a history of childhood sexual abuse. She denied any current alcohol or recreational drug use. Her family members described her as "moody" and "extremely self-critical and manipulative," although history gathered from them was limited, as Ms. J would not allow the treating team to contact them after initial collateral was gathered. The nursing home staff described her as "difficult and uncooperative," stating that she was intermittently non-adherent with both psychiatric and systemic medical treatments, including coumadin that she was on for atrial fibrillation. The nursing home staff described "splitting" behavior by this patient, stating that she would fluctuate between idealizing and devaluing different staff members as "good" and "bad" staff. She repeatedly requested extra doses of opiates and coumadin, stating she wanted to die by euthanasia. After multiple threats to hoard her pills and overdose if she was not moved to a different room at the nursing home, concern over suicidal ideation precipitated her admission to the psychiatric inpatient unit.

During her inpatient stay, the splitting behavior continued with multiple complaints about certain "bad" nursing staff and fluctuating degrees of adherence to care depending on who was working with her. She made multiple complaints about trivial issues, displayed anger when her needs were not met immediately, and repeatedly complained about her children not visiting and not inviting her to live with them. She repeatedly stated that she "felt isolated and abandoned" by her children despite their report that they were frequently present figures in the patient's life, but that it was impossible to ever meet all of her excessive expectations. Ms. J demonstrated frequent mood changes, easily provoked emotional outbursts that were intense and out of proportion to the circumstances, and irritability in response to perceived slights or insults. She continued to report transient and intermittent thoughts of self-harm, telling staff she was planning to roll down the stairs in her wheelchair. When asked about prior requests for euthanasia, Ms. J stated that she had made these threats because she desperately wanted to move rooms at the nursing home as she was in a quadruple room and simply wanted more privacy. Based on the clinical symptoms observed and collateral longitudinal history of frantic efforts to avoid abandonment, unstable and intense interpersonal relationships, recurrent suicidal behavior, marked reactivity of mood, and disproportionate displays of intense anger, a diagnosis of BPD was made.

Case 2 – Ms. P

Ms. P, a 74-year-old widowed mother of three children, was admitted for alcohol withdrawal requiring medical monitoring given a history of alcohol withdrawal seizures. After medical clearance on the medicine unit, she was transferred to the geriatric psychiatry inpatient unit for further assessment of her safety due to a number of suicidal statements she had made to the medical team. She had a past psychiatric history of an unspecified depressive disorder, thought to be secondary to an alcohol use disorder. She had a history of binge-purging behavior throughout her 30s and 40s without ever meeting formal diagnostic criteria for an eating disorder. She also reported a history of experimentation with various substances throughout her adult life but alcohol was her substance of choice. She continued to drink alcohol in a weekend binge pattern, typically 500 ml or more of distilled spirits in 24 hours. She had a past medical history of hypertension, pancreatitis, and alcohol withdrawal seizures. She was widowed for 15 years and estranged from each of her three children. She described a history of verbal and emotional abuse by her mother and an absent father.

Collateral history from her outpatient primary care physician and psychiatrist indicated that this patient often presented as emotionally labile or "moody" in that she had a short temper with intermittent bouts of rage. Her primary care physician, who had known the patient for over 20 years, stated that she demonstrated excessive interpersonal sensitivity and seemed to be "easily offended" or "slighted". He stated that this patient frequently ended up in the emergency room when he was away on vacation with vague somatic complaints, alcohol withdrawal, or suicidal ideation. Her primary care physician stated that she had abused alcohol intermittently for years despite negative consequences including prior pancreatitis and a driving under the influence charge.

While on the geriatric psychiatry inpatient unit, various staff members observed irritable, depressive, and hostile behavior. She repeatedly threatened to report or sue certain nursing staff whom she had deemed "incompetent". Throughout her stay, and particularly in times of distress, she would threaten suicide stating that she was going to starve herself to death or cut herself. She would fluctuate between threatening to decline benzodiazepines as a preventative treatment for alcohol withdrawal seizures as per the revised Clinical Institute Withdrawal Assessment for Alcohol (CIWA-Ar) scale [14] and demanding that nursing staff give her more than the prescribed amount. Several staff members developed hostile reactions to Ms. P, expressing frustration and anger when having to care for her. Certain staff members felt valued and as though they could build rapport while others felt degraded and condescended to when interacting with her. Based on the clinical observations and collateral longitudinal history from her primary care physician of unstable and intense interpersonal relationships, impulsivity leading to self-damaging behaviors, recurrent suicidal behavior, marked reactivity of mood, and disproportionate displays of anger, a diagnosis of BPD was made.

PSYCHOMETRIC RATING SCALES

There is a lack of age-adjusted screening or diagnostic tools to assess BPD in the geriatric population. One of the more commonly used tools is the Diagnostic Interview for Borderlines-Revised (DIB-R) [15, 16]. The Zanarini Rating Scale for Borderline Personality Disorder (ZAN-BPD) is a clinician administered scale used to assess change in BPD symptoms over time [17]. Despite the fact that these tools align with many of the DSM diagnostic criteria for BPD, they do not account for age-related changes such as cognitive impairment, or other medical and psychiatric comorbidities [12]. When assessing older adult patients with suspected BPD, it is also important to rule out possible comorbidities. Depression should be routinely screened for particularly in institutional settings including medical inpatient units and nursing home facilities. Such screening tools include the Geriatric Depression Scale (GDS) [18] or the Brief Assessment Schedule for the Elderly (BASDEC) [19]. Harmful or hazardous drinking can be identified by the Alcohol Related Problems Survey (ARPS), although this screening tool was developed for use in older adult patients in a primary care setting [20]. The CAGE and Michigan Alcoholism Screening Test - Geriatric Version (MAST-G) have been validated for use in older adults including in an inpatient setting [21]. Cognitive status can be determined using the Montreal Cognitive Assessment (MoCA) [22]. For further information on psychometric instruments, refer to Chapter 6.

BARRIERS TO DIAGNOSIS

There are many barriers that exist in the accurate and timely diagnosis of BPD in the older adult population, particularly in institutional settings. There is an inconsistent diagnostic process that exists for this cohort of patients with some clinicians applying BPD criteria "loosely", while others subjectively change individual criteria to what they think may be more appropriate to a geriatric population. One of the main issues can be the lack of an accurate and thorough longitudinal history demonstrating the pervasive and chronic nature of borderline traits. Barriers to diagnosis are summarized in Figure 4-2. To further illustrate this, barriers to diagnosis for Ms. J included underlying mild neurocognitive impairment, suspected substance misuse, and patient refusal for contact of family for collateral information. Barriers to diagnosis for Ms. P included lack of longitudinal informants other than her primary care physician and the diagnostic difficulty given her chronic alcohol misuse and the effect this substance had on her mood and interpersonal relationships.

Specific stressors related to old age including persistent illness/ impairment, demographic changes including moving to a nursing home facility or unemployment/retirement, and losses secondary to death or disability can also contribute to difficulty in establishing the degree to which patterns of unstable interpersonal relationships exist [12]. Moreover, a number of confounding issues can mask underlying symptoms of BPD, such as comorbid psychiatric or systemic medical conditions, frailty, or medication side effects causing an individual to appear less impulsive than they actually are. For example, both Ms. J and Ms. P may have presented as less impulsive secondary to their chronic opioid and alcohol use, respectively. Similarly, certain symptoms of BPD such as impulsivity or irritability can resemble the clinical presentation of other disorders more often seen in a geriatric population such as a major or mild frontotemporal neurocognitive disorder, or the cumulative effects of substance abuse or suicide attempts (e.g., by overdose) on cognitive status.

KEY POINTS: CLINICAL DIAGNOSIS

- The DSM criteria for BPD may lack face validity in the elderly population.
- Affect dysregulation, inappropriate and chronic anger, and feelings of emptiness tend to be relatively stable over time and therefore more common in the older adult BPD population.
- Impulsivity and self-harming behaviors tend to decrease in intensity as a patient ages.
- Certain behaviors may simply transform over time such as self-injurious behaviors manifesting as food or hydration refusal, medication non-adherence, and general actions that sabotage medical care.
- There is a lack of age-adjusted screening or diagnostic screening tools for diagnosing BPD in the older adult population.
- Barriers to diagnosis include lack of longitudinal history as a result of biased positive recall in patients, cognitive impairment in the patient and/or co-informants, lack of co-informants, or co-informants with little knowledge of the patient's earlier life.

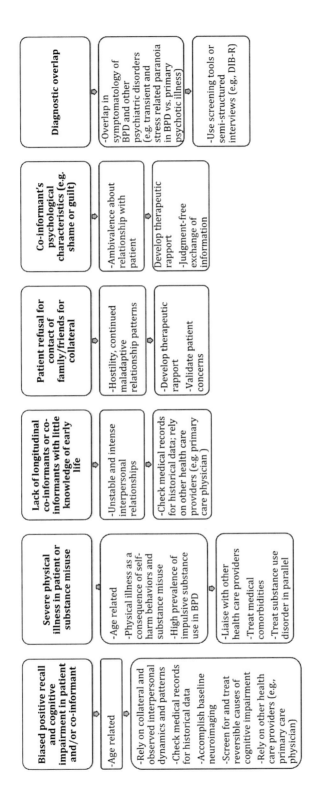

Figure 4-2. Barriers to Diagnosing Borderline Personality Disorder in Older Adults.

REFERENCES

[1] Personality disorders. *Diagnostic and Statistical Manual of Mental Disorders. Text Revision.* 4th ed. Washington, DC: American Psychiatric Association; 2000: 706-710.

[2] Personality disorders. *Diagnostic and Statistical Manual of Mental Disorders.* 5th ed. Arlington, VA: American Psychiatric Publishing; 2013: 766-767.

[3] Oltmanns TF, Balsis S. Personality Disorders in Later Life: Questions about the measurement, course, and impact of disorders. *Annu Rev Clin Psychol.* 2011; 7: 321-349.

[4] Galione JN, Oltmanns TF. The relationship between borderline personality disorder and major depression in later life: Acute versus temperamental symptoms. *Am J Geriatr Psychiatry.* 2013; 21(8): 747-756.

[5] Zanarini MC, Frankenburg FR, Hennen J, Silk KR. The longitudinal course of borderline psychopathology: 6-year prospective follow-up of the phenomenology of borderline personality disorder. *Am J Psychiatry.* 2003; 160(2): 274-283.

[6] Arens EA, Stopsack M, Spitzer C, et al. Borderline Personality Disorder in Four Different Age Groups: A cross-sectional study of community residents in Germany. *J Pers Disord.* 2013; 27(2): 196-207.

[7] Trappler B, Backfield J. Clinical characteristics of older psychiatric inpatients with borderline personality disorder. *Psychiatry Q.* 2001; 72(1): 29-40.

[8] Hunt M. Borderline personality across the life span. In: Malatesta V. *Mental Health Issues of Older Women: A Comprehensive Review for Health Care Professionals.* Binghamton, NY: The Haworth Press Inc; 2007: 173-191.

[9] Stevenson J, Meares R, Comerford A. Diminished impulsivity in older patients with borderline personality disorder. *Am J Psychiatry.* 2003; 160(1): 165-166.

[10] Rosowsky E, Gurian B. Borderline personality disorder in late life. *Int Psychogeriatr.* 1991; 3(1): 39-52.

[11] Rosowsky E, Gurian B. Impact of borderline personality disorder in late life on systems of care. *Hosp Community Psychiatry.* 1992; 43(4): 386-389.

[12] Agronin ME, Maletta G. Personality disorders in late life. Understanding and overcoming the gap in research. *Am J Geriatr Psychiatry.* 2000; 8(1): 4-18.

[13] Welleford EA, Harkins SW, Taylor JR. Personality change in dementia of the Alzheimer's type: relations to caregiver personality and burden. *Exp Aging Res.* 1995; 21(3): 295-314.

[14] Sullivan JT, Sykora K, Schneiderman J, Naanjo CA, Sellers EM. Assessment of alcohol withdrawal: the revised clinical institute withdrawal assessment for alcohol scale (CIWA-Ar). *Br J Addict.* 1989; 84(11): 1353-1357.

[15] Zanarini MC, Gunderson JG, Frankenburg FR, Chauncey DL. The revised diagnostic interview for borderlines: discriminating BPD from other Axis II disorders. *J Pers Disord.* 1989; 3: 10-18.

[16] Gunderson JG, Kolb JE, Austin V. The diagnostic interview for borderline patients. *Am J Psychiatry.* 1981; 138(7): 896-903.

[17] Zanarini MC, Vujanovic AA, Parachini EA, Boulanger JL, Frankenburg FR, Hennen J. Zanarini Rating Scale for Borderline Personality Disorder (ZAN-BPD): a continuous measure of DSM-IV borderline psychopathology. *J Pers Disord.* 2003; 17(3): 233-242.

[18] Yesavage JA, Brink TL, Rose TL, et al. Development and validation of a geriatric depression screening scale: A preliminary report. *J Psychiatr Res.* 1982-1983; 17: 37-49.

[19] Adshead F, Cody DD, Pitt B. BASDEC: a novel screening instrument for depression in elderly medical inpatients. *BMJ.* 1992; 305(6850): 397.

[20] Fink A, Morton SC, Beck JC, et al. The alcohol-related problems survey identifying hazardous and harmful drinking in older primary care patients. *J Am Geriatr Soc.* 2002; 50(10): 1717-1722.

[21] Sorocco KH, Ferrell SW. Alcohol use among older adults. *J Gen Psychol.* 2006; 133(4): 453-467.

[22] Nasreddine ZS, Phillips NA, Bedirian V, et al. The Montreal Cognitive Assessment, MoCA: a brief screening tool for mild cognitive impairment. *J Am Geriatr Soc.* 2005; 53(4): 695-699.

Chapter 5

COMORBIDITIES IN BORDERLINE PERSONALITY DISORDER: ROLE OF CONSULTATION AND COLLABORATION

Glen L. Xiong[1,], MD, CMD,*
Tricia K. W. Woo[2], MD, MSc,
and Mariam Abdurrahman[3], MD, MSc

[1]Health Sciences Associate Clinical Professor, Psychiatry
Department of Psychiatry and Behavioral Sciences
University of California, at Davis, CA, US
[2]Associate Professor, Division of Geriatric Medicine, Department of Medicine,
Michael G. DeGroote School of Medicine, Faculty of Health Sciences,
McMaster University, Hamilton, ON, Canada
[3]Department of Psychiatry and Behavioural Neurosciences,
Michael G. DeGroote School of Medicine, Faculty of Health Sciences,
McMaster University, Hamilton, ON, Canada

Borderline personality disorder (BPD) is known to complicate the treatment of chronic psychiatric disorders, especially treatment-refractory depression. It is also highly comorbid with bipolar disorder, posttraumatic stress disorder, and substance use disorders. As older adults are more likely to suffer from systemic medical conditions, BPD can also complicate the treatment of such medical conditions, especially the chronic pain leading to misuse of prescription opioid pain medication, increased medical morbidity, and worse functional outcomes.

INTRODUCTION

As stated elsewhere in the book, there are no reliable prevalence estimates for geriatric BPD, but in the general population this is estimated to be 1.4-1.8% [1, 2]. BPD is associated

---

*Corresponding author: glen.xiong@ucdmc.ucdavis.edu.

with a high degree of functional impairment and a 10% risk of mortality in 10 years [3, 4]. BPD has a high rate of comorbidities with mood disorders and substance use disorders, and is associated with a high degree of mental health service utilization. BPD is also hypothesized to be an important predictor of major health problems and worse general medical outcomes [5]. This chapter reviews the array of psychiatric, systemic medical and neurocognitive comorbidities (See Figure 5-1) in older adults with BPD, and the role of psychiatrists as consultants and collaborators.

PSYCHIATRIC COMORBIDITIES

There is a considerable overlap between the core features of BPD and bipolar and major depressive disorders which may make precise differential diagnoses difficult [6]. BPD commonly leads to secondary major depressive disorder and to treatment resistance. Remission of major depressive disorder does not necessarily predict remission in BPD, although remission of major depressive disorder is more often preceded by prior improvement in BPD [7, 8]. The high frequency of diagnostic co-occurrence and resemblance of phenomenological features has led some authors to suggest that BPD is part of the bipolar spectrum [9-10]. Posttraumatic stress disorder also shares several core features with BPD, including interpersonal dysfunction and affective instability. In a study by Shea et al. [11], 68% of patients with posttraumatic stress disorder also met diagnostic criteria for BPD. There is also strong evidence to support the high comorbidity between substance use disorders and BPD [12]. To complicate this further, patients with BPD and bipolar disorder may have a higher risk of substance use disorder, compared to those with bipolar disorder alone [13]. We describe below the increasing recognition of BPD and misuse of opioid pain medications.

SYSTEMIC MEDICAL COMORBIDITIES

As the incidence of systemic illness increases with age, there may be a significant impact on health outcomes in older adults with BPD. Among community-dwelling adults, BPD is associated with a greater likelihood of having serious systemic medical conditions including cardiovascular disease, stroke and hypertension [14, 15]. One recent study by Powers and Oltmanns [16] used interviewer, self and informant report of personality pathology and found that BPD features were related to the presence of obesity and arthritis. Even subthreshold symptoms of BPD seemed to be predictive of serious systemic health risks.

Borderline pathology may be an important adverse health risk as people age. Individuals with BPD appear to be at increased risk of obesity, obesity-related conditions, such as back pain and diabetes, and syndromic conditions, such as fibromyalgia, chronic fatigue and temporomandibular joint syndrome [17]. Furthermore, in the McLean Study of Adult Development (MSAD), remissions of BPD were associated with a significantly reduced likelihood of having the preceding medical conditions [17-19]. During a 10-year prospective follow-up period, MSAD [20] also detected a significant association between increases in cumulative body mass index and the following variables: self-harm, dissociation, and a number of socio-demographic correlates such as being single, having a low income, being on disability, being rated as having a fair to poor Global Assessment of Functioning score, and having a poor occupational or academic history. Therefore, BPD may serve as a link between psychosocial risk factors and increased body mass index and obesity.

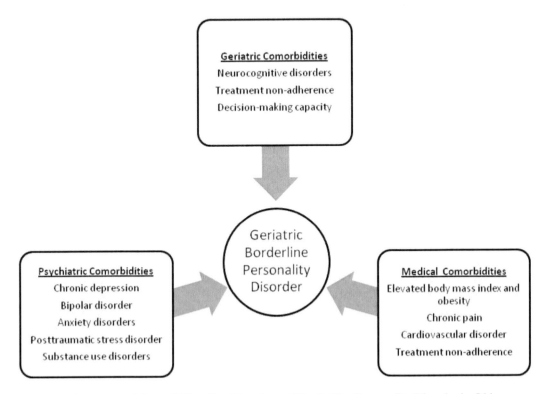

Figure 5-1. Summary of Comorbidity Considerations of Borderline Personality Disorder in Older Adults.

As mentioned above, BPD is associated with substance use disorders and has received increasing attention as a risk factor for prescription opioid medication misuse. In a study with participants between the ages of 18 and 52 years (mean age 20.39 years), BPD was associated with greater quantity and frequency of opioid use, risk for pain medication misuse, and opioid dependence [21]. The key BPD features of self-harm and impulsivity appeared to account for opioid misuse [21]. In a general adult outpatient clinic, men with BPD were also most likely to misuse pain medication including mixing prescribed pain medications for recreational purposes [22]. As most of the studies on BPD and prescription pain medication misuse currently focus on the general adult populations, more research is needed in geriatric BPD with chronic pain and use of opioid pain medications.

Although substance use disorders constitutes one of the leading causes of disability worldwide, substance use is often underappreciated in the care of older adults [23]. Since the number of older adults continues to increase because of cohort changes, the public health impact of substance use disorders will likely amplify. This will inexorably involve the aging patients with BPD with comorbid substance use disorders. Increasing demands on the substance abuse treatment centers will require development of effective service programs to address the needs of the aging drug-using population, including those with personality disorders. Finally, as older adults with chronic pain are increasingly seeking treatments in specialized pain clinics, it is likely that pain clinics will either have to develop their own expertise in psychiatric and substance abuse treatment or collaborate actively with psychiatrists and other mental health professionals.

NEUROCOGNITIVE COMORBIDITIES AND OTHER CONSIDERATIONS IN OLDER ADULTS

In older adults there is much higher prevalence of neurocognitive disorders and changes in personality may be among the earliest signs for Alzheimer's type [18] and frontotemporal neurocognitive disorders [24]. This raises further questions regarding the possibility that personality may be associated with the impact of aging on brain structures. There are overlaps in frontotemporal neurocognitive disorder and BPD symptoms and in at least one case report that posed significant diagnostic dilemmas [25]. Finally, as individuals with neurocognitive disorders are more likely to regress to earlier stages of coping, BPD features may also emerge in the elderly even though they may not meet the full BPD criteria. Such features commonly include impulsivity, affective instability, and excessive anger. In institutional settings, the consulting psychiatrist is often called to assist the primary medical team in distinguishing the etiology of disruptive behavioral problems in older adults with neurocognitive disorders and borderline features, and implement effective treatment plans. While often challenging to differentiate, both neurocognitive disorders and BPD affect an individual's ability to understand their medical conditions, manipulate information, and carry out Activities of Daily Living (ADLs)—therefore leading to problems with treatment adherence and decision-making capacity. The ability to recognize BPD that is superimposed on neurocognitive disorder is paramount to management since some aspects of BPD (e.g., emotional lability and impulsivity) may be "reversible" when they are appropriately contained and treated.

ROLE OF PSYCHIATRIC CONSULTATION AND COLLABORATION

Indeed it is critical for psychiatrists to recognize and diagnose BPD in older adult patients. These patients are most likely to be referred to psychiatrists for:

- chronic depression
- treatment non-adherence
- opioid pain medication misuse
- assessment of medical decision-making capacity (Also see Chapter 9 on decision-making capacity).

Since BPD in older adults present differently than in middle age, there is a higher likelihood that BPD is missed in older adults (See Chapter 4 on clinical diagnosis of BPD). Psychiatrists can play a key role in terms of clarifying the needs of the geriatric patients with BPD and also collaborate with other clinicians to co-manage and develop comprehensive treatment approaches. Older adults with BPD may still show the typical vacillation between overvaluing and demeaning care providers and family caregivers. This can lead to considerable frustration on the part of caregivers as well as staff. Patients with BPD may have self-harming behaviors such as non-adherence to therapy or even active sabotage of medical care. Himelick and Walsh [26] reviewed BPD pathology in long-term care settings and pointed out some of these types of experiences and made recommendations for care providers on how to develop intervention strategies. The emphasis was placed on validating the BPD patient's needs while encouraging caregiver staff to set up appropriate boundaries. Actual losses associated with aging may also trigger decompensation in older patients with BPD. Normal fear of abandonment may be exaggerated in BPD patients and this may lead to demanding and antagonistic behavior with caregivers.

The consulting psychiatrist can play a critical role by helping other clinicians recognize their own countertransference reactions and thereby still provide effective and empathic treatments for the geriatric patient with BPD. The traditional consultation-liaison model has evolved into integrated and collaborative care models. For integrated models, mental health professionals may co-locate and work with primary care providers to provide on-site comprehensive care by the primary care provider, psychiatrist and social worker, during a single visit to the clinic. Collaborative care models take various forms and generally involve a team-based approach, where care managers coordinate care among key clinician team members (usually involving primary care provider, social worker, and psychiatrist). Under this collaborative model, psychiatrists serve as educators about BPD and lead team-based treatment approaches. The burgeoning integrative and collaborative care models will likely increase the impact that psychiatrists make in the well-being of older adults with BPD, especially in institutional settings.

The following is a case description, in order to illustrate and summarize some of the difficulties the specialists in institutional settings may encounter when caring for aging patients with comorbid BPD.

Case – Ms. A

Ms. A, a 68-year-old female with diabetes mellitus, chronic obstructive pulmonary disease, chronic pain, and morbid obesity and hypertension, was diagnosed with BPD in her early 30s. She was twice divorced and was estranged from her daughter. She lived alone in a house and was independent for her activities of daily living. Her diagnosis of BPD was confirmed by a geriatric psychiatrist and she had been undergoing psychotherapy with cognitive behavioral emphasis for the previous 5 years. Ms. A was compliant with general medical treatment until one year before presentation when she was admitted to hospital with an exacerbation of her chronic obstructive pulmonary disease due to medication non-adherence. She responded well to medical therapy and was discharged after two weeks with a course of oral prednisone. Once home, she declined all her community supports and alienated all those charged with her care. She declined to resume cognitive behavioral therapy and would not allow her daughter to visit. She discontinued her prednisone and was non-adherent to her diabetic diet. She declined physically and after two months was readmitted to acute care hospital. During her hospitalization, she would frequently complain of severe diffuse pain in her lower extremities and headaches. The primary medical team continued her maintenance opioid pain medications and had been increasing the dose without any evidence of improvement. They consulted the psychiatric and pain management teams.

The psychiatric team interviewed Ms. A and recognized that she had a history of BPD and were able to establish rapport with her by discussing her prior treatments for borderline personality, identify major progress that she made during treatment with her outpatient mental health provider, and validating her current concerns and feeling of hopelessness about her multiple medical problems. Ms. A noted that she had been having much more difficulty with the fact that she did not get along with her daughter and was fearful that Ms. A may die before they make amends. Because of this, she had not been interested in managing her medical problems. She was able to recognize that she was having much more emotional pain than physical pain. While she had fantasized that her medical doctors would call her daughter and tell the daughter that Ms. A was going to die soon so that the daughter would come and visit, she acknowledged that it was best that she called her daughter herself after she left the hospital and continued follow-up with her outpatient providers.

KEY POINTS: COMORBIDITIES IN BORDERLINE PERSONALITY DISORDER: ROLE OF CONSULTATION AND COLLABORATION

- BPD is highly comorbid with mood, anxiety and substance use disorders, and is likely a major unrecognized risk factor for obesity and cardiovascular disease.
- The misuse of prescription pain medications and treatment of chronic pain in older adults is an emerging area of interest, and attention to borderline personality pathology is warranted.
- BPD in older adults should be considered when psychiatrists are consulted about chronic depression, treatment non-adherence, opioid pain medication misuse, and decision-making capacity.
- Symptoms of BPD in older adults have considerable impact on systemic medical disorders for geriatric patients who may also have neurocognitive disorder—leading to problems with treatment adherence and medical decision making.
- Psychiatrists have traditionally play consultative roles and are increasingly taking part in integrative and collaborative care models, especially in institutional settings.

REFERENCES

[1] Swartz M, Blazer D, George L, Winfield I. Estimating the prevalence of borderline personality disorder in the community. *J Pers Disord.* 1990; 4(3): 257-272.

[2] Grant BF, Chou CP, Goldstein RB, et al. Prevalence, correlates, disability, and comorbidity of DSM-IV borderline personality disorder: results from the wave 2 national epidemiologic survey on alcohol and related conditions. *J Clin Psychiatry.* 2008; 69(4): 533-545.

[3] Zimmerman M, Chelminski I, Young D, Dalrymple K, Martinez J, Morgan TA. Which DSM IV personality disorders are most strongly linked with indices of psychosocial morbidity in psychiatric outpatients? *Compr Psychiatry.* 2012; 53(7): 940-945.

[4]   Paris J. Chronic suicidality among patients with borderline personality disorder. *Psychiatr Serv.* 2002; 53(6); 738-742.

[5]   Bender DS, Dolan RT, Skodol, et al. Treatment utilization by patients with personality disorders. *Am J Psychiatry.* 2001; 158(2): 295-302.

[6]   Smith DJ, Muir WJ, Blackwood DH. Is borderline personality disorder part of the bipolar spectrum? *Harv Rev Psychiatry.* 2004; 12(3): 133-139.

[7]   Gunderson JG, Morey LC, Stout RL, et al. Major depressive disorder and borderline personality disorder revisited: longitudinal interactions. *J Clin Psychiatry.* 2004; 65(8): 1049-1056.

[8]   Leichsenring F, Leibing E, Kruse J, New AS, Leweke F. Borderline personality disorder. *Lancet.* 2011; 377(9759): 74-84.

[9]   Zimmerman M, Morgan TA. The relationship between borderline personality disorder and bipolar disorder. *Dialogues Clin Neurosci.* 2013; 15(2): 155-169.

[10] Balsis S, Lowmaster S, Cooper LD, Benge JF. Personality disorder diagnostic thresholds correspond to different levels of latent pathology. *J Pers Disord.* 2011; 25(1): 115-127.

[11] Shea MT, Zlotnick, C, Weisberg RB. Commonality and specificity of personality disorder profiles in subjects with trauma histories. *J Pers Disord.* 1999; 13(3): 199-210.

[12] Trull TJ, Sher KJ, Minks-Brown C, Durbin J, Burr R. Borderline personality disorder and substance use disorders: A review and integration. *Clin Psychol Rev.* 2000; 20(2): 235-253.

[13] Hidalgo-Mazzei D, Walsh E, Rosenstein L, Zimmerman M. Comorbid bipolar disorder and borderline personality disorder and substance use disorder. *J Nerv Ment Dis.* 2015; 203(1): 54-57.

[14] Lee HB, Bienvenu OJ, Cho S-J, et al. Personality disorders and traits as predictors of incident cardiovascular disease: Findings from the 23-year follow-up of the Baltimore ECA study. *Psychosomatics.* 2010; 51(4): 289-296.

[15] Moran P, Stewart R, Brugha T, et al. Personality disorder and cardiovascular disease: Results from a national household survey. *J Clin Psychiatry.* 2007; 68(1): 69-74.

[16] Powers AD, Oltmanns TF. Borderline personality pathology and chronic health problems in later adulthood: The mediating role of obesity. *Personal Disord.* 2013; 4(2): 152-159.

[17] Zanarini MC. Diagnostic specificity and long-term prospective course of borderline personality disorder. *Psychiatr Ann.* 2012; 42(2): 53-58.

[18] Frankenburg FR, Zanarini MC. The association between borderline personality disorder and chronic medical illnesses, poor health related lifestyle choices, and costly forms of health care utilization. *J Clin Psychiatry.* 2004; 65(12): 1660-1665.

[19] Zanarini MC, Frankenburg FR, Hennen J, Reich DB, Silk KR. Prediction of the 10-year course of borderline personality disorder. *Am J Psychiatry.* 2006; 163(5): 827–832.

[20] Frankenburg FR, Zanarini MC. Relationship between cumulative BMI and symptomatic, psychosocial, and medical outcomes in patients with borderline personality disorder. *J Pers Disord.* 2011; 25(4): 421-431.

[21] Tragesser SL, Jones RE, Robinson RJ, Stutler A, Stewart A. Borderline personality disorder features and risk for prescription opioid use disorders. *J Pers Disord.* 2013; 27(4): 427-441.

[22] Sansone RA, Watts DA, Wiederman MW. The misuse of prescription pain medication and borderline personality symptomatology. *J Opioid Manag.* 2013; 9(4): 275-279.

[23] Oslin DW. Evidence-based treatment of geriatric substance abuse. *Psychiatr Clin North Am.* 2005; 28(4): 897-911.

[24] Rankin KP, Baldwin E, Pace-Savitsky C, Kramer JH, Miller BL. Self awareness and personality change in dementia. *J Neurol Neurosurg Psychiatry.* 2005;76(5): 632-639.

[25] Salzbrenner LS, Brown J, Hart G, et al. Frontotemporal dementia complicated by comorbid borderline personality disorder: a case report. *Psychiatry (Edgmont).* 2009; 6(4): 28-31.

[26] Himelick AJ, Walsh J. Nursing home residents with borderline personality traits: Clinical social work interventions. *J Gerontol Soc Work.* 2002; 37(1): 49-63.

In: Borderline Personality Disorder in Older Adults
Editors: A. Hategan, J. A. Bourgeois, G. L. Xiong

ISBN: 978-1-63482-221-3
© 2015 Nova Science Publishers, Inc.

Chapter 6

PSYCHOLOGICAL ASSESSMENT OF BORDERLINE PERSONALITY DISORDER IN GERIATRIC PATIENTS

Jelena P. King[1,2,3,*], PhD, CPsych,
Christina B. Gojmerac[1,2,4], PhD, CPsych
and Heather E. McNeely[1,2,3], PhD, CPsych
[1]Department of Psychiatry and Behavioural Neurosciences,
McMaster University, Hamilton, ON, Canada
[2]Clinical Neuropsychology Service, St. Joseph's Healthcare Hamilton,
Hamilton, ON, Canada
[3]Schizophrenia & Community Integration Service,
St. Joseph's Healthcare Hamilton, Hamilton, ON, Canada
[4]Seniors Mental Health Program, St. Joseph's Healthcare Hamilton,
Hamilton, ON, Canada

Psychological assessment to diagnose borderline personality disorder (BPD) in geriatric patients requires adaptation and consideration of age-related factors that impact assessment and interpretation, and differs from the approach taken with younger individuals. Psychological assessments need to be sensitive to age-graded differences because BPD in geriatric individuals can be clinically different compared to younger adults. This poses significant challenges with respect to the current diagnostic nosology and psychological measures available to diagnose BPD in geriatric individuals. In this chapter, recommendations and practical approaches to manage these challenges will be provided. Highlighted are two self-report personality measurement tools valid across the age span and recommended for use in geriatric BPD screening.

* Corresponding author: kingj@stjoes.ca.

INTRODUCTION

When geriatric patients suspected of BPD present in clinical settings, psychological assessment is often necessary to assist with diagnosis, treatment and management. BPD symptoms in geriatric patients often differ from those characterized earlier in life. Morgan et al. [1] compared young and older adults with BPD with respect to psychiatric comorbidity, frequency of specific BDP criteria and functional impairment in a variety of domains. While older BPD adults were less likely to endorse impulsivity, self-harm, and affective instability, they reported greater life-time hospitalizations and a higher degree of interpersonal impairment. These findings suggest BPD symptoms might change over time, but functional ability continues to be significantly impacted; findings broadly consistent with other research demonstrating age-related attenuation in some BPD symptoms but pervasive, extensive and relatively more stable functional impairment [2, 3].

This poses challenges for accurate assessment with respect to reliability, validity, and the utility of currently available clinical measures [4]. It might be necessary to assess for less prototypic BPD features in geriatric patients to avoid overlooking the disorder if over-reliance is placed on the symptoms classically associated with BPD presentation in younger individuals. For example, probing more carefully to assess the degree of social isolation secondary to pervasive deficits in interpersonal functioning rather than focusing on symptoms of impulsivity or self-harm. An assessment approach modified to focus less on strict application of current Diagnostic and Statistical Manual (DSM-5) criteria and more on dimensional measurement of BPD traits is likely more appropriate.

Clinical measures assessing symptoms of BPD are often tied to context that is more applicable to younger individuals. DSM criteria require demonstration that maladaptive personality patterns impair social and occupational functioning; however, challenges are presented in determining when the threshold for functional impairment has been reached for geriatric patients who are retired, never worked outside the home, or have smaller social networks [5]. Additionally, geriatric individuals often experience significant changes in life circumstances such as death-related loss of support, difficulties adjusting to retirement, or medically-related physical decline. This introduces the additional challenge of establishing whether functional difficulties reflect an exacerbation of BPD symptoms or an appropriate, time-limited response to a psychosocial stressor or life transition. In this vein, the issue of context within our current diagnostic nosology and how it relates to geriatric BPD symptoms can be more complex and difficult to untangle.

Conditions such as mild or major neurocognitive disorder/dementia, delirium or physiological reactions to medication changes can contribute to behavioral disturbance and affective instability that could be interpreted as a personality disorder. These issues are magnified in psychiatric inpatient settings where patients frequently present with comorbid psychiatric illness, cognitive difficulties, and poorly treated medical problems. These complexities often warrant multiple assessment measures and methods (including a combination of medical investigations, cognitive testing, and collateral informants) to determine whether the behavioral disturbance reflects a medical condition or are more pervasive and longstanding and consistent with BPD.

PSYCHOLOGICAL ASSESSMENT APPROACH

Personality Assessment to Assist Diagnosis

In psychiatric settings, patients often present with personality traits that might be maladaptive in certain contexts and put them at risk for developing comorbid psychiatric disorders. The rates of co-occurrence between BPD and major depressive disorder in geriatric patients are just as high as in younger adults [6] and associated with amplified functional deficits, illness chronicity, and treatment challenges [7, 8]. In this vein, knowledge of an individual's personality architecture and determining whether traits are consistent with BPD can greatly assist in diagnosis and treatment planning.

Psychological Screening Measures

When the patient has been medically stabilized there may be comorbid psychiatric diagnoses, and chronic medical conditions that can reduce stamina, interfere with valid response style and contribute to the exacerbation of BPD traits during testing. In these instances, administration of a lengthy diagnostic interview (such as the Structured Clinical Interview for DSM Disorders) may not be the best starting point. Rather, self-report measures that simultaneously screen for comorbid psychiatric disorders, personality architecture, and validity of responding would be the recommended first line approach. A screening measure could then inform lengthier structured diagnostic investigation. Implementing psychological screening measures before embarking on more time consuming structured clinical interviews has empirical support. While self-report measures might yield higher base rates of criteria endorsement in BPD evaluations [9-11], they are not necessarily less valid than diagnostic interviews and a combined use of these methods optimally identifies BPD [12].

Several self-report psychological measures are available for BPD assessment (reviewed in 7); however, the majority of these have either not been validated in geriatric populations or they were underrepresented in the normative samples. Consequently, these measures may have uncertain reliability and validity to accurately detect BPD in older adults [7] and accordingly, they should be used cautiously and in conjunction with multiple measures and methods. In contrast, those select measures that have been validated in geriatric populations are listed in Figure 6-1 [7, 13-18]; two of which will be reviewed in greater detail.

Personality Assessment Inventory (PAI)

The PAI [13] has been validated in geriatric populations with age-appropriate normative data and good generalizability making it a favorable choice as a geriatric BPD screening measure. It is a self-administered, objective inventory of adult personality that is designed to provide information relevant to clinical diagnosis of major psychiatric (including personality) disorders, treatment planning, and screening for psychopathology. The 344 PAI items comprise 22 non-overlapping scales (4 validity, 11 clinical, 5 treatment, and 2 interpersonal). Most relevant to screening for BPD are the validity scales and the Borderline Features (BOR) scale. Four validity scales assessing factors that could distort self-report are recommended as the starting point to determine whether the individual is responding honestly and consistently, and not over or under-reporting symptoms to an extent that would invalidate test results. The BOR scale consists of 24 statements querying an individual's stability of mood, self-image, identity confusion and self-worth, intense and unstable interpersonal relationships, impulsivity, and self-harm. These questions produce a total scale (BOR) and four subscale scores that comprise different elements of BPD presentation. Research has shown that the PAI-BOR discriminates reasonably well between BPD patients and those with major depressive disorder or dysthymia and is measurement invariant across sex and age [19].

The PAI can be used as a screening instrument when BPD is suspected in geriatric individuals to determine whether more structured assessment is required. Providing the patient has a 4th grade reading level and sufficient stamina to complete the questionnaire, it can often be completed in less than one hour. Recommended accommodations include: breaking the test into several sessions for those experiencing fatigue; reading items aloud or using audiotaped versions for individuals with reduced visual acuity; clinician recording of responses for patients with reduced fine motor control or pain; and clarification of items for those with mild neurocognitive disorder.

Personality Assessment Inventory (PAI; 13)

NEO Personality Inventory-Revised (NEO-PI-R; 14)

Minnesota Multiphasic Personality Inventory-2 (MMPI-2; 15)

International Personality Disorders Examination (IPDE; 16)

Structured Clinical Interview for DSM–IV Axis II Personality Disorders (SCID-II; 17)

Structured Interview for DSM–IV Personality (SIDP-IV; 18)

Figure 6-1. Psychological Measures to Assess Personality Disorders Validated in Normative Samples of Older Adults (adapted from 7).

Revised NEO Personality Inventory (NEO-PI-R)

This 240-item self-report questionnaire assesses five broad domains of personality (Neuroticism, Extraversion, Openness, Agreeableness, and Conscientiousness) as conceptualized by the Five Factor Model of personality [14]. Each broad domain subsumes several more specific traits or "facets" that capture more unique personality information [20]. The NEO-PI-R is one of the few self-report tools that measure personality traits equally well across the lifespan [21, 22], and younger and older adults with the same position on a personality trait of interest endorse the majority of NEO-PI-R items similarly [23]. A large scale review [24] of the association between DSM personality disorders and the Five Factor Model showed that BPD patients tend to score high on neuroticism and low on agreeableness and conscientiousness, findings which have been confirmed in two meta-analyses [25, 26].

Case – Ms. A

Ms. A, a 70-year-old divorced woman, was admitted to hospital due to behavioral difficulties at her long-term residential care home. Once medically stabilized, she was referred for psychological evaluation, with query regarding BPD. Psychological assessment was completed over numerous brief sessions due to fatigue secondary to chronic back pain related to rheumatoid arthritis. During an initial unstructured interview, Ms. A was uncertain of the purpose of her hospitalization and stated it may have been because she had been "crying a lot and emotional" virtually every day, something she felt was related to poor medical management of her chronic pain. However, she admitted to feeling increasingly emotional because she did not get to see her family enough. She denied any discord with staff or co-residents and was unaware of any complaints that had been made against her. Collateral information obtained from her three daughters revealed that Ms. A had a history of depression and longstanding "emotional ups and downs" related to hypersensitivity and interpersonal difficulties. In the weeks leading up to her hospitalization, she had expressed to them being "desperate for help" because she felt her needs were not being met. There had been some interpersonal events with staff in the home where she was reprimanded for "crossing boundaries" with some co-residents, and going into their rooms uninvited. During visits, her daughters perceived Ms. A as initially happy, before "digressing into self-pity mode" at which point she would express grievances regarding her treatment at the home and anger at her daughters and ex-husband for abandoning her. Her daughters corroborated Ms. A's reports of severe arthritis pain and its negative impact on both her mood and interpersonal functioning.

During the psychological evaluation, three emotional triggers were identified: (1) feelings of being mistreated and misunderstood by staff, (2) feelings of abandonment by her family, and (3) her chronic pain. These were recurring themes throughout the evaluation even when they were not being directly queried and her responses were often tangential in the direction of these topics. Adjustments were made to minimize Ms. A's pain by allowing her to lie down while she listened to the examiner read the questions from the PAI and NEO-PI-R and record her responses for her. Structured Clinical Interviews for DSM were administered after PAI results indicated adequate validity of responding and elevations on depression and borderline scales.

The assessment revealed primary diagnoses of recurrent major depressive disorder, and BPD. Ms. A's psychiatric difficulties were felt to be severe and complicated by a longstanding and pervasive personality style that included emotional lability, chronic feelings of emptiness, poor sense of self, untrustworthiness in relationships, and pervasive impairment in interpersonal functioning. These aspects of her personality were felt to increase her risk of recurrent major depressive episodes in the context of significant arthritis pain. Ms. A's associated perception of mistreatment with respect to pain management, along with the actual physical discomfort, served to exacerbate those aspects of her personality architecture that were unappealing and disagreeable. Recommendations were provided to her treatment team to be mindful of the link between her physical and psychological pain, and not attribute her challenging interpersonal style as a fundamental character flaw.

KEY POINTS: PSYCHOLOGICAL ASSESSMENT OF BORDERLINE PERSONALITY DISORDER IN GERIATRIC PATIENTS

- Start with psychological screening measures validated in geriatric populations that provide information regarding the validity of self-report and the presence of BPD features. Accommodations for fatigue, physical limitations, or mild cognitive impairment may be required.
- If screening measures indicate valid response style and elevations on BPD scales, Structured Clinical Interviews for DSM Disorders are recommended, including evaluation for other psychiatric illness(es) due to strong comorbidity between BPD and other disorders.
- Collateral informants are recommended to ascertain the longitudinal course of potential BPD, and degree and pervasiveness of functional impairment.
- Personality testing using the NEO-PI-R dimensional approach is recommended to identify personality architecture that could inform the appropriateness of certain therapeutic modalities to assist treatment planning.

REFERENCES

[1]   Morgan TA, Chelminski I, Young D, Dalrymple K, Zimmerman M. Differences between older and younger adults with borderline personality disorder on clinical presentation and impairment. *J Psychiatr Res.* 2013; 47(10): 1507-1513.

[2]   Drake RI, Vaillant GE. Longitudinal views of personality disorder. *J Pers Disord.* 1988; 2: 44-48.

[3]   Trappler B, Backfield J. Clinical characteristics of older psychiatric inpatients with borderline personality disorder. *Psychiatr Q.* 2011; 72(1): 29-40.

[4]   Oltmanns TF, Balsis S. Personality disorders in later life: questions about the measurement, course, and impact of disorder. *Annu Rev Clin Psychol.* 2011; 7: 321-349.

[5]   Segal DL, Hersen M, Van Hasselt B, Silberman CS, Roth L. Diagnosis and assessment of personality disorder in older adults: A critical review. *J Pers Disord.* 1996; 10: 384-399.

[6]   Morse JQ, Lynch TR. Personality disorders in late life. *Curr Psychiatry Rep.* 2000; 2(1): 24-31.

[7]   Zweig RA. Personality disorder in older adults: assessment challenges and strategies. *Prof Psychol Res Pr.* 2008; 39(3): 298-305.

[8]   Galione JN, Oltmanns TF. The relationship between borderline personality disorder and major depression in later life: acute versus temperamental symptoms. *Am J Geriatr Psychiatry.* 2013; 21(8): 747-756.

[9]   Hunt C, Andrews G. Measuring personality disorder: The use of self-report questionnaires. *J Pers Disord.* 1992; 6(2): 125-133.

[10] Hyler SE, Skodol AE, Kellman HD, Oldham JM, Rosnick L. Validity of Personality Diagnostic Questionnaire-Revised: Comparison with two structured interviews. *Am J Psychiatry.* 1990; 147(8): 1043-1048.

[11] Hyler SE, Skodol AE, Oldham JM, Kellman HD, Doidge N. Validity of the Personality Diagnostic Questionnaire-Revised: A replication in an outpatient sample. *Compr Psychiatry.* 1992; 33(2): 73-77.

[12] Hopwood CJ, Morey LC, Edelen MO, Shea MT, Grilo CM, Sanislow CA, McGlashan TH, Daversa MT, Gunderson JG, Zanarini MC, Markowitz JC, Skodol AE. A comparison of interview and self-report methods for the assessment of borderline personality disorder criteria. *Psychol Assess.* 2008; 20(1): 81-85.

[13] Morey LC. *The Personality Assessment Inventory: Professional manual.* Odessa, FL: Psychological Assessment Resources, 1991.

[14] Costa PT, Jr, McCrae RR. *Professional manual: Revised NEO Personality Inventory (NEO-PI-R) and NEO Five Factor Inventory (NEO-FFI).* Odessa: Psychological Assessment Resources, 1992.

[15] Butcher JN, Dahlstrom WG, Graham JR, Tellegen A, Kaemer B. *Minnesota Multiphasic Personality Inventory-2 (MMPI-2): Manual for administration and scoring.* Minneapolis, MN: University of Minnesota Press, 1989.

[16] World Health Organization. *The International Personality Disorder Examination (IPDE) DSM-IV Module.* Washington, DC: American Psychiatric Association Press, 1995.

[17] First MB, Gibbon M, Spitzer RL, Williams JB, Benjamin LS. *Structured Clinical Interview for DSM-IV Axis II Personality Disorders (SCID-II).* Washington, DC: American Psychiatric Association Press, 1997.

[18] Pfohl B, Blum N, Zimmerman M. *Structured Interview for DSM-IV Personality (SIDP-IV).* Iowa City: University of Iowa, 1995.

[19] De Moor MH, Distel MA, Trull TJ, Boomsma DI. Assessment of borderline personality disorder features in population samples: Is the Personality Assessment Inventory-Borderline Features scale measurement invariant across sex and age? *Psychol Assess* 2009; 21(1): 125-130.

[20] Soto CJ, John OP, Gosling SD, Potter J. Age differences in personality traits from 10 to 65: Big five domains and facets in a large cross-sectional sample. *J Pers Soc Psychol* 2011; 100(2): 330-348.

[21] Costa PT Jr, McCrae RR. Personality stability and its implications for clinical psychology. *Clin Psychol Rev.* 1986; 6(5): 407-423.

[22] McCrae RR, Costa PT Jr. Validation of the five-factor model of personality across instruments and observers. *J Pers Soc Psychol.* 1987; 52(1): 81-90.

[23] Van den Broeck J, Rossi G, Dierckx E, De Clercq B. Age-neutrality of the NEO-PI-R: Potential differential item functioning in older versus younger adults. *J Psychopathol Behav Assess.* 2012; 34(3): 361-369.

[24] Widiger TA, Costa PT. Five-factor model personality disorder research. In: Costa, PT, Widiger, TA, eds. *Personality Disorders and the Five Factor Model of Personality,* 2nd ed. Washington, DC: American Psychological Association; 2002: 59-87.

[25] Saulsman LM, Page AC. The five-factor model and personality disorder empirical literature: A meta-analytic review. *Clin Psychol Rev.* 2004; 23(8): 1055-1085.

[26] Samuel DB, Widiger TA. A meta-analytic review of the relationship between the five-factor model and DSM-IV-TR personality disorders: A facet level analysis. *Clin Psychol Rev.* 2008; 28(8): 1326-1342.

SECTION III

MANAGEMENT

In: Borderline Personality Disorder in Older Adults
Editors: A. Hategan, J. A. Bourgeois, G. L. Xiong

ISBN: 978-1-63482-221-3
© 2015 Nova Science Publishers, Inc.

Chapter 7

THERAPEUTIC ALLIANCE AND BOUNDARY ISSUES

Usha Parthasarathi[1],, MBBS and Brian Holoyda[2], MD, MPH*

[1]Associate Clinical Professor of Psychiatry, Department of Psychiatry and Behavioural
Neurosciences, Michael G. DeGroote School of Medicine, Faculty of Health Sciences,
McMaster University, Hamilton, ON, Canada
[2]Psychiatry Resident, University of California,
Davis Medical Center, Sacramento, CA, US

Therapeutic alliance is a negotiated collaboration between two parties, the clinician and the patient, and is the foundation on which a working relationship is developed. The strength and the quality of the therapeutic alliance do much to determine the clinical outcome. Therapeutic alliance is developed on the basis of trust between two individuals and it can be predictably challenging to establish a therapeutic alliance with patients suffering from borderline personality disorder (BPD). By the nature of their symptomatology, including interpersonal difficulties and cognitive distortions, patients with BPD can also present as a medico-legal challenge for a clinician. In this chapter, we explain the concept of therapeutic alliance, benefits of therapeutic alliance, ways to establish and maintain the therapeutic alliance in patients with BPD, understand therapeutic alliance rupture and how to re-establish therapeutic alliance following the rupture. Common medico-legal challenges in patients in BPD and methods to safeguard and manage these challenges will also be described.

INTRODUCTION

"The quality of the therapeutic alliance is the most robust predictor of outcome" –
Safran & Muran [1].

The essential components of therapeutic alliance are bonds, goals, and tasks. Therapeutic alliance develops on a therapeutic *bond* that is based on mutual trust, acceptance and confidence. A strong working alliance is characterized by jointly developed *goals* (or

---

* Corresponding author: uparthas@stjoes.ca.

outcomes) that are the target of the therapeutic intervention. *Tasks* are the means to achieve the goals. Tasks should be perceived as relevant and efficacious and the clinician and the patient must accept responsibility to collaborate in order to achieve the tasks [2, 3]. Positive therapeutic alliance is not, in and of itself, curative; rather, the working alliance is seen as the ingredient that "makes it possible for the patient to accept and adhere to treatment faithfully" [2-6].

As discussed in previous chapters, BPD is characterized by pronounced affective and cognitive disturbances, interpersonal disruption, and impulsive behavior. Dysfunctional behaviors and transference and countertransference processes contribute to numerous challenges in establishing therapeutic alliance in a patient with BPD [7, 8]. Patients with BPD present with self-regulation difficulties, self-destructive behavior and can assume the role of victim. These behaviors may invoke (in an otherwise calm and self-confident clinician) strong feelings of hostility, guilt, fear, doubt, inadequacy, and helplessness. Clinicians may view these patients as help-rejecting complainers, and may avoid seeing them all together and may find themselves saying or doing things that would be atypical for them in usual clinical practice [7-9].

THERAPEUTIC CONTRACTING IN MANAGEMENT OF BORDERLINE PERSONALITY DISORDER IN OLDER ADULTS

Research suggests that development of a strong therapeutic alliance in a patient with BPD is essential for effective intervention [7, 8]. There are several methods by which therapeutic alliance can be established, with therapeutic contracting having the most empirical evidence to support its efficacy in establishing and maintaining therapeutic alliance in patients with BPD [7, 8, 10, 11]. The therapeutic contract is a formal written negotiated agreement between the patient and the clinician. Each aspect of day-to-day care of the patient is considered for the negotiation; the goals and the objectives of the contract are clearly defined and agreed to by both the parties [8, 10, 11]. By virtue of the negotiation and agreement, the contract is collaborative in nature and helps to decrease the "power imbalance" that a patient may experience. With the therapeutic contract, the aim is to create a safe and predictable treatment environment and to involve the patient in their own care and recovery. The use of the therapeutic contract facilitates therapeutic alliance and may help in containment of dangerous behavior, such as excessive aggression and acting out; it provides integrity to the treatment plan and helps to stabilize transference and countertransference; and it has been described as the fulcrum between the clinician and the patient [10]. The therapeutic contract can be particularly useful for management of patients in residential and institutional settings such as hospitals, nursing homes and retirement homes [10]. Clear identification of a patient's goals and objectives, explanation of the responsibilities and duties of the clinician towards the patient, and description of the patient's expected behavior and predictable methods for appropriate limit setting should be included in the therapeutic contract [10, 11]. A negotiated decrease in self-harm or treatment-sabotaging behavior itself can save a patient's life. In older borderline patients, clinical scenarios where therapeutic alliance may be especially important include optimization of medical workups, avoidance of possibly dangerous procedures and medications, and self-management for surveillance for medication side effects.

Miller [11] identified the following principles for a successful therapeutic contract for an inpatient or another institutional setting:

- The contract should begin with a clear statement of purpose of treatment mutually agreed upon by the patient and staff.
- The purpose of the treatment should be defined in terms of concrete goals that are realistically achievable during the course of inpatient or institution stay, as the case may be.
- The body of the contract should clearly specify the responsibility of the patient and the staff. It should also clearly state what can and cannot be realistically provided by the staff.
- Consequences in terms of positive or negative reinforcers for a behavioral intervention should be discussed with the patient and clearly stated in the contract.
- If the therapeutic contract requires patient to stop using previous dysfunctional mechanisms (e.g., starving, medication non-adherence, acting out or self-harm) it should explicitly provide for alternative methods of coping (e.g., listening to music, journaling, walking away, talking to friends and family, knitting). The contract should allow the patient to taper, rather than suddenly discontinue maladaptive patterns.
- The contract should be developed as a joint effort of the patient and the treatment team, and sometimes the patient's family or significant others.
- Once the contract is signed, copies should be readily available to the patient and to all the staff.
- Consistency in the implementation of the therapeutic contract by all the staff is essential to the success of the contract.

Miller [11] also identified common errors in formulating a therapeutic contract, such as contracts used as a substitute for therapeutic conversation, for covert punishment or rejection of the patient by the clinical team, or the contract providing false sense of security leading to neglect of impending risks. These errors arise from being either unduly restrictive or overly paternalistic. A formal contract is effective only as an adjunct to other treatment modalities; there should always be an attempt to understand the reasons for a particular behavior in a patient instead of relying solely on the contract agreement to manage behavior. Table 7-1 describes a sample of a therapeutic contract.

FACTORS THAT INFLUENCE THE THERAPEUTIC ALLIANCE

Patients with BPD engage in behaviors that can often be destructive to the therapeutic alliance. Allen [8] explained the sequence of how therapeutic alliance breaks down and how the process can be frustrating to a clinical team. He stated that when persistently confronted by the troublesome acting-out behavior characteristic of the patient with BPD, clinicians may feel angry, used, abused, unappreciated, unreasonably attacked, disempowered, guilty about not being able to relieve the patient's suffering, or anxious about the ramifications of the patient's symptoms.

Table 7-1. Sample of Therapeutic Contract for Patient: *Ms. X*

> *Ms. X* and the treatment team realize that, when *Ms. X*'s hope is reawakened by a new treatment situation, *she* becomes terrified of reliving past disappointments. *Ms. X* protects *herself* by _____ (starving/self-harm acts/treatment refusal/getting angry/withdrawing, etc.). *Ms. X* has no experience with other reliable methods of self-protection or self-soothing and has difficulty noticing early signs of anxiety. The _____ (starving/self-harm acts/treatment refusal/getting angry/withdrawing, etc.) produce temporary relief but long-term guilt and lowered self-esteem.
>
> **To address this problem, *Ms. X* and the clinical treatment team agree to the following contract:**
>
> **Goal:** To decrease and then eliminate _____ (starving/self-harm acts/treatment refusal/getting angry/withdrawing, etc.) and replace them with effective, safe means of anxiety reduction.
>
> **Terms:**
> - *Ms. X* agrees to write a list of at least ten alternatives to _____ (starving/self-harm acts/treatment refusal/getting angry/withdrawing, etc.) and to try these, one by one, until effective ones are found. Staff agrees to assist in generating and testing these ideas.
> - Staff agrees to assist *Ms. X* in identifying early signs of anxiety and anger. *Ms. X* will list these and practice recognizing them. *Ms. X* will monitor *her* feelings and behavior in a journal.
> - *Ms. X* agrees to notify staff of impending _____ (starving/self-harm acts/treatment refusal/getting angry/withdrawing, etc.). Staff agrees to be available when approached for this purpose. For each day *she* succeeds at this, *Ms. X* will be able to access _____ of (half-hour trip to the library with staff/*herself*, listening to music/1:1 time for 1 hour with the staff, choosing the music playlist, etc.) which *she* has identified as a meaningful privilege to help *her* motivation.
> - While *Ms. X* and the staff agree to collaborate to maintain everyone's safety, all recognize that _____ (starving/self-harm acts/treatment refusal/getting angry/withdrawing, etc.) is unlikely to be fully eliminated immediately. However, clear progressive decrease is expected; e.g., no more than one _____ (starving/self-harm acts/treatment refusal/getting angry/withdrawing, etc.) incident per day for the next week, no more than two self-harm incidents during the following week, and then no _____ (starving/self-harm acts/treatment refusal/getting angry/withdrawing, etc.) incidents.
> - If _____ (starving/self-harm acts/treatment refusal/getting angry/withdrawing, etc.) do occur, the usual consequences of aggressive behavior will follow, using the least restrictive alternative that is effective to maintain safety.
> - Staff agrees to provide opportunities for safe discussion of difficult feelings. If *Ms. X* feels unsafe, *she* will inform staff, who will help restore a feeling of safety.
> - It is recognized by *Ms. X* and the treatment team that *Ms. X* is frightened of progress and recovery. It is the joint responsibility of the patient and staff to maintain this as the active focus of treatment.
> - *Ms. X* and the treatment team will meet daily to evaluate progress. Any recommended modifications of this contract can be discussed at those meetings.
>
>   **Time Period for the Contract:** _____ (3 days, 2 weeks, etc.)
>   **Next Date of Review:**
>   **Ten identified alternative safer methods to cope with distress:**
>   **Signed by** *Dr. Psychiatrist* **Signed by** *Mr. Staff* **Signed by** *Ms. X*

(Adapted from Miller, 1990; 11).

Anxiety caused by a sense of guilt, inadequacy, helplessness, or frustration might lead clinician to look for ways to make a patient feel better quickly, even in the face of help-rejecting responses by the patient. A clinician might reluctantly indulge the patient's unreasonable demands out of a sense of pity, a wish to placate the patient, or a misguided hope of ridding themselves of the problem. When these efforts fail, the patient might become even more critical and negativistic toward the clinician. This sequence can induce a problematic behavior in the clinician such as hostility towards patient or blaming and criticizing the patient for unreasonable behavior. Hostility might be overt, in the form of mean-spirited personal attacks, or subtle, in the form of pathologizing patients by making pejorative attributions, or for geriatric patients, describing them as being memory-impaired and unable to make decisions. This may also lead to a clinician accusing the patient of being unaware of the damage he or she is causing - a subtle accusation of lack of intelligence - by pointing out the obvious or lecturing the patient. A disrupted therapeutic alliance can negatively affect the therapeutic milieu and the patient might be abandoned with a permanent rupture of the therapeutic alliance.

Allen [8] also identified techniques to manage these disruptive behaviors. Clinicians are encouraged to think of these methods when managing a difficult interaction with a patient with BPD. Being mindful of patient's state of mind and having a consistent approach can often help in sustaining and improving therapeutic alliance. A few practical tips to engage patients with BPD in therapeutic relationships are described in Figure 7-1 [8, 9, 11-13]. For illustrating some common disruptive behaviors displayed by older patients with BPD and methods to manage them, see Figure 7-2.

- Any clinician interaction with the patient should model on interpersonal respect. Respectful treatment of the patient by clinicians in the face of the patient's chaotic behavior may help the patient modify their behavior (9, 11, 12).

- Clinicians should present themselves as comfortable with their own limitations and unwilling to make unusual or risky interventions. Clinicians should present as unafraid of patient's anger, neediness or anxiety, and be unwilling to attack the patient in the face of provocation (11, 12).

- The best way to avoid transference/countertransference problems is to keep firm boundaries – both physical and verbal. No matter how hurtful the verbal attacks or how seductive the offers from the patient may be, the clinician should remain empathic, calm, friendly and stick to the terms of the therapeutic contract (8, 9, 13).

- Clinicians should be honest in their interactions with patients and they should agree clearly on what they are able to offer and what their limitations are (9).

- Clinicians should also recognize mistakes and errors happen. Mistakes can be used to therapeutic advantage; clinicians should openly admit the mistake without undue defensiveness, lengthy explanations, or request for forgiveness (9, 13).

Figure 7-1. Practical tips to engage patients with borderline personality disorder in therapeutic relationships.

Patient's response	Clinician's response	Case scenario
• Patient makes seemingly dramatic and excessive accusations against the clinician or significant others or voices highly exaggerated pronouncements.	• Clinician attempts to find the kernel of truth in the statement or the reaction and validate it, while ignoring the hyperbole.	• Ms. X, 66 years old, angrily says to Dr. P, "What would you understand what I go through with my children. My children hate me. You are young and rich, what would you understand!" Dr. P uses calm voice and reflects back, "Yes, I am young but, I appreciate how much pain you are in. I am here to help you. I know you are very upset and I want to help you make sense of this pain".
• Patient refuses to eat or drink.	• Clinician views patient as reasonable and her behavior as negotiable.	• The clinical team reduced Ms. X's lorazepam from 1 mg/day to 0.75 mg/day the previous day despite the patient's resistance to medication change. The next day Ms. X went on a hunger strike to protest the "injustice" and stated, "Anyway, I am just waiting to die, so who cares?!" Nurse N meets with Ms. X in a quiet place and says, "You must have a good reason for choosing to starve. I also know you must be hungry and you are certainly not enjoying this. I am concerned for you. I am sure we can find a way to better solution, you do not have to go through suffering from hunger".
• Patient constantly asks clinicians for "extra help" and loudly demanding immediate relief.	• Clinician should be honest with the patients regarding their own limitations. Clinician should make a straightforward statement about what he or she may or may not be able to do, calmly but unapologetically.	• Ms. X says to Nurse A, "I am so weak, I cannot even get up from bed. Sweetie, can you clean my feet in the bed?" Nurse A is aware that Ms. X's primary nurse has already spoken to Ms. X earlier that day and had informed her that Ms. X was expected to attend to her foot care independently. Nurse A calmly states to Ms. X that the team expects Ms. X to attend to her foot care independently and therefore, she will not be available to help her with the foot care.
• Patient attempts to embroil the clinician in disputes.	• Clinician should be approachable and validate any kernels of truth in patient's concerns but a clinician should avoid both direct involvement and "taking sides" by pointing out to the patient that clinician does not have enough information on what happened to make an objective judgement about it.	• Ms. X approaches Dr. P and says, "Dr. O did not know what he was doing, he gave me a low quality implants in my hip. I am in so much pain since this replacement. I am depressed and traumatized by my operation. I want to sue him, Dr. P can you talk to my lawyer and tell him about how Dr. O ruined my life. You know how much I am suffering". Dr. P listens calmly to Ms. X's request and says, "I know you are distressed by your situation. However, I am not in a position to comment on Dr. O's contribution to the situation". "Would you like to speak to Dr. O directly?"

Figure 7-2. Common Disruptive Behaviors and Practical Management Approaches for Geriatric Borderline Personality Disorder.

BOUNDARIES AND MEDICO-LEGAL ISSUES

From a legal standpoint, the physician-patient relationship is fiduciary, or based on "the inherent necessity for trust and confidence" requiring "scrupulous good faith on the part of the physician" [14]. The fiduciary nature of the relationship between the clinician and the patient is presumed, but orienting the treatment frame to foster and maintain appropriate boundaries that promote trust can be difficult. Patients with BPD are at high risk for psychological distress from boundary violations; therefore, the clinicians should exercise caution when treating them [15]. Though conducting treatment in a legally appropriate manner may seem intuitive, there are other aspects of the treatment that, if established early, can reduce the risk of boundary violations in the treatment of patients with BPD.

The most common malpractice claims brought against physicians treating patients with BPD are suicide and sexual misconduct [16]. As older patients are at risk of becoming victims of "elder abuse," geriatric patients with BPD may in fact perceive their clinicians in a negative way, such that they may accuse clinicians of being abusive. The accusations are frequently made against nursing staff rather than physicians, although psychiatrists are frequently called upon to investigate such claims of "abuse."

Addressing some basic legal principles in treatment can prevent boundary violations that may occur in the course of a clinician's relationship with a patient with BPD. Basic components of the treatment frame such as treatment setting, duration of treatment (in-session and longitudinally), fees, and no-show policy should all be established at the outset of therapy and, to the greatest degree possible, adhered to during the course of the patient's treatment. Patients with BPD may attempt to alter the frame, requesting to be seen in a different setting or for a longer period of time. The clinician should be aware of countertransference issues that may draw for him or her to make such alterations and remain cognizant of the message he or she communicates when making such accommodations. Such changes may lead to boundary crossings and boundary violations that could cause psychological distress to patients with BPD. Sexual exploitation of or sexual intercourse with any patient is illegal and ethically indefensible. A clinician who engages in such behavior can be sued for negligence and sexual misconduct. Typically, such behaviors are preceded by progressive boundary violations [17].

Another important element of the patient's treatment is confidentiality, which the clinician must maintain except under specific clinical and legal circumstances. The clinician should inform the patient about the limits of confidentiality, preferably at the outset of treatment, to prevent ruptures in the therapeutic relationship if the need to violate the patient's confidentiality arises [18]. For example, a clinician may break confidentiality if a patient is at imminent danger of harming her/himself or harming another or if there is suspected child abuse occurring in the patient's home. For patients with BPD who commonly experience chronic suicidal ideation and inappropriate anger that can manifest in threats against others' lives, it is critical that the clinician educates the patient about the limits of confidentiality.

Informed consent, a legal necessity to provide treatment and procedures to patients, consists of informing a patient of the risks, benefits, and alternatives to treatment and ensuring that the patient's choice is communicated freely and in accordance with his or her wishes. It has been posited that BPD patients who do not understand their treatment choices and associated risks may blame the therapist for treatment that the patients believe may be of a lower standard [16, 18]. Engaging patients in discussions of informed consent maintains autonomy, which may be a therapeutic goal for a patient with BPD with dependency needs, and promotes the therapeutic alliance.

KEY POINTS: THERAPEUTIC ALLIANCE AND BOUNDARY ISSUES

- Therapeutic alliance is an important factor in any clinical outcome; establishing and maintaining therapeutic alliance with patients with BPD can be challenging, however, there are many effective methods by which a therapeutic relationship can be established with patients with BPD.
- Honesty, respect, understanding, kindness and consistency from the staff can help overcome common disruptive issues that are inherent in a therapeutic relationship with a patient with BPD.
- When treating patients with BPD, a clinician should be aware of boundary issues to safeguard themselves from boundary violations.

REFERENCES

[1]   Safran JD, Muran JC. *Negotiating the therapeutic alliance: a relational treatment guide*: Guilford Press; 2000.

[2]   Bordin E. The generalizability of the psychoanalytic concept of the working alliance. *Psychotherapy*. 1979; 16(3): 252-260.

[3]   Dryden W, Reeves A. *Key issues for counselling in action*. SAGE publications Ltd; 2008.

[4]   Piper WE, Ogrodniczuk JS, Lamarche C, Hilscher T, Joyce AS. Level of alliance, pattern of alliance, and outcome in short-term group therapy. *Int J Group Psychother.* 2005; 55(4): 527-550.

[5]   Barber JP, Connolly MB, Crits-Christoph P, Gladis L, Siqueland L. Alliance predicts patients' outcome beyond in-treatment change in symptoms. *J Consult Clin Psychol.* 2000; 68(6): 1027-1032.

[6]   Castonguay LG, Constantino MJ, Holtforth MG. The working alliance: Where are we and where should we go? *Psychotherapy (Chic).* 2006; 43(3): 271-279.

[7]   Gabbard GO. An overview of countertransference with borderline patients. *J Psychother Pract Res.* 1993; 2(1): 7-18.

[8]   Allen DM. Techniques for reducing therapy-interfering behavior in patients with borderline personality disorder. Similarities in four diverse treatment paradigms. *J Psychother Pract Res.* 1997; 6(1): 25-35.

[9]   Richardson-Vejlgaard R, Broudy C, Brodsky B, Fertuck E, Stanley B. Predictors of psychotherapy alliance in borderline personality disorder. *Psychother Res.* 2013; 23(5): 539-546.

[10] Bloom H, Rosenbluth M. The use of contracts in the inpatient treatment of the borderline personality disorder. *Psychiatr Q.* 1989; 60(4): 317-327.

[11] Miller LJ. The formal treatment contract in the inpatient management of borderline personality disorder. *Hosp Community Psychiatry.* 1990; 41(9): 985-987.

[12] Siefert CJ. A goal-oriented limited-duration approach for borderline personality disorder during brief inpatient hospitalizations. *Psychotherapy (Chic).* 2012; 49(4): 502-518.

[13] Benjamin LS. *Interpersonal reconstructive therapy, an integrative, personality-based treatment for complex cases.* Guilford Press; 2006.

[14] Omer v. Edgren. *38 Wash. App.* 376, 685 P.2d 635 (1984).

[15] Gutheil T. Patients involved in sexual misconduct with therapists: is a victim profile possible? *Psychiatr Ann.* 1991; 21(11): 661-667.

[16] Simon R. Treatment of boundary violations: clinical, ethical, and legal considerations. *Bull Am Acad Psychiatry Law.* 1992; 20(3): 269-288.

[17] Simon R. Sexual exploitation of patients: How it begins before it happens. *Psychiatr Ann.* 1989; 19(2): 104-112.

[18] Gutheil TG. Medicolegal pitfalls in the treatment of borderline patients. *Am J Psychiatry.* 1985; 142(1): 9-14.

In: Borderline Personality Disorder in Older Adults   ISBN: 978-1-63482-221-3
Editors: A. Hategan, J. A. Bourgeois, G. L. Xiong   © 2015 Nova Science Publishers, Inc.

Chapter 8

SUICIDALITY IN GERIATRIC BORDERLINE PERSONALITY DISORDER: CLINICAL APPROACHES AND MANAGEMENT

Jessica E. Waserman[1,], MD, Karen Saperson[2], MBChB,*
Christina B. Gojmerac[3], PhD, CPsych
and Christine Stanzlik-Elliott[4], MSW

[1]Psychiatry Resident, Department of Psychiatry and Behavioural Neurosciences,
Michael G. DeGroote School of Medicine, Faculty of Health Sciences,
McMaster University, Hamilton, ON, Canada
[2]Associate Professor, Psychiatry, Associate Chair of Education,
Department of Psychiatry and Behavioural Neurosciences,
Academic Head of Division of Geriatric Psychiatry,
Michael G. DeGroote School of Medicine, Faculty of Health Sciences,
McMaster University, Hamilton, ON, Canada
[3]Clinical Psychologist, Department of Psychiatry and Behavioural Neurosciences,
Michael G. DeGroote School of Medicine, Faculty of Health Sciences,
McMaster University, Hamilton, ON, Canada
[4]Discharge Specialist, St. Joseph's Healthcare Hamilton,
Hamilton, ON, Canada

A significant complication of borderline personality disorder (BPD) is a range of self-damaging suicidal behaviors, including deliberate non-suicidal self-harm, suicide attempts, and deaths by suicide. This chapter discusses suicidality in the geriatric BPD population. The authors review the dynamics and clinical presentation of suicidality in this group, and summarize the clinical approaches to assessment and management of these patients, particularly in institutional settings.

---

* Corresponding author: jessica.waserman@medportal.ca.

INTRODUCTION

The significant burden of BPD is perhaps most evident in its high mortality rate due to suicide, as 60-70% of patients with BPD will attempt suicide throughout the course of their illness, and 5-10% will take their own lives [1]. This rate is almost 50 times higher than that of the general population [1]. The geriatric population carries an additional high risk for suicide, particularly the subset of older males [2]. Although the BPD population is predominantly female, most BPD patients who complete suicide are male [3, 4]. As older age and BPD are both risk factors for suicide, older adults with BPD can be considered an especially high-risk group.

Those with BPD often lack the adaptive coping skills and social support networks needed to face the aging process and its attendant losses, role transitions and dependency. The population with BPD is particularly vulnerable to the stressor of transitioning to an institutional setting, where feelings of abandonment often intensify, and where there are externally imposed behavioral routines and social interactions, often at odds with individual preferences.

Clinicians have few evidence-informed guidelines to direct care and improve quality of life, and are left feeling vulnerable to medico-legal risks. Both the conditions of aging and BPD are often plagued by stigma in the health care system, posing yet another barrier to accessing services and treatment. This section provides a clinical approach to the risk assessment of suicide in geriatric patients with BPD. We discuss the etiology, risk and protective factors, and special considerations and management strategies for geriatric BPD patients with suicide in a variety of treatment settings.

DEFINITION OF TERMS

A helpful set of definitions used to describe the spectrum of self-harming behaviors was put forth by the American Psychiatric Association in their practice guidelines for suicidal patients [5]. Usage of consistent terminology for the spectrum of self-harming behaviors can facilitate communication and minimize confusion among clinicians, researchers, public health practitioners, and patients.

Deliberate self-harm is defined as willful self-infliction of painful, destructive or injurious acts without the intent to die. As described in one of the core criteria of DSM-5 [6], patients with BPD are characterized by "recurrent suicidal behavior, gestures, or threats, or self-mutilating behavior." Suicidality in patients with BPD tends to be of a more chronic nature, whereas suicidality associated with mood disorders, for example, may present acutely during a mood episode.

Individuals with BPD often exhibit recurrent suicide attempts emerging in adolescence, and continuing into late adulthood. The intensity of suicidal ideation and behavior may wax and wane over time, depending on life stressors. However, these behaviors tend to decrease over time or merely manifest differently [7], as illustrated in the following case scenario. Difficulties in establishing a diagnosis of BPD in late life may reflect alterations in the environmental and social context, such that core symptoms may manifest differently [8] (e.g., self-harm may manifest as willful food refusal). This alteration in clinical presentation is important to recognize within acute and long-term care delivery systems, as it can facilitate adaptation of service provision to enhance the care of geriatric patients with BPD.

Case – Mrs. B, "The Challenging Patient"

Mrs. B, a cachectic 83-year-old, was living in a nursing home for one year prior to presentation. She had been admitted to the nursing home following a hip fracture that compromised her mobility, as her husband was unable to care for her at home.

Mrs. B had led a somewhat chaotic life, characterized by marked interpersonal difficulties and repeated disappointment in others. She constantly criticized her two adult daughters and husband for not visiting and not caring for her sufficiently, although the family generally visited daily in the evenings. If they missed a visit, she would sob, refuse her meals, medications, and personal care, and threaten to kill herself. Her care team often became concerned about dehydration due to her intermittent refusal of oral intake. She argued with her daughters when they did visit, demanding that they intervene with the facility's administrators to address her multiple concerns. At other times, she was jovial, denied any suicidal thoughts, and appeared content with her living situation.

In a family meeting with the facility's social worker, the daughters reported that prior to admission, Mrs. B's husband was overwhelmed and exhausted by her demands. They indicated that their parents' marriage had always been fraught with explosive arguments initiated by their mother. They recalled several occasions throughout her life where Mrs. B threatened suicide in the context of family conflicts, and one occasion where she overdosed on medication in their presence. They described their mother as extremely sensitive to perceived criticism, resulting in her termination from various jobs as a legal secretary, despite being bright and competent.

Mrs. B's pattern of relating to others was replicated with the long-term care staff. She would insult and demean the staff, making comments about their race, appearance and cultural background. She often became verbally and physically aggressive in the context of personal care. She also pitted staff against each other, initiating rumors and gossip about alternating team members. She endorsed the staff were "mean" to her, and favored other residents over her. Despite her disdain for them, she often tried to keep caregivers in her room by making numerous requests. Team members were uncomfortable around Mrs. B, and tried to avoid being assigned to provide her care. Because of a pervasive pattern of marked mood reactivity, unstable and intense interpersonal relationships, recurrent suicidal behavior, and frantic efforts to avoid abandonment, a diagnosis of BPD was eventually made, whereas an acute mood episode was ruled out. Subsequently, a suicide risk assessment was completed and a management plan was implemented by the health care team.

Clinical care teams in various institutional settings may often experience situations when older patients present with challenging interpersonal dynamics and management dilemmas, as seen in Mrs. B's case. A few practical tips regarding the management of such patients in a long-term care setting, many of which may also be adapted to other institutional settings, are illustrated in Figure 8-1.

> *Consistency is Key:*
> - The health care team should be educated about characteristic behaviors and interpersonal dynamics seen in BPD, to minimize personalization.
> - Consistent caregivers are preferable to rotating staff, to ensure consistent behavioral responses and boundaries between caregiver and patient.
> - A written care plan posted in the patient's room is helpful for team members, and in addition provides a sense of comfort to the individual, signifying that they are not being abandoned.
> - Staff should maintain consistent behavioral responses to verbal aggression; e.g., leave the room and allow the individual to calm down.
> - Staff should be instructed to redirect and disengage when the individual engages in splitting of team members; e.g., "I prefer not to listen to complaints about my colleague. Let's focus on how we can help you today".
> - Family members should also be encouraged and supported to set appropriate limits.

Figure 8-1. Helpful Tips for Managing Borderline Personality Disorder in Institutional Settings.

UNDERSTANDING THE CAUSES OF SUICIDE IN BORDERLINE PERSONALITY DISORDER

The etiology of suicidal behavior is difficult to study and there are few theoretical models that explain suicide in general or specific to BPD and older adults. One recently proposed theory has attempted to do so. According to the Interpersonal Theory of Suicide by Van Orden et al. [9], suicide results from an increased *desire for suicide* (driven by feelings of thwarted belongingness and the perception of burdensomeness) combined with an acquired *capability for suicide* (via increased physical pain tolerance and/or reduced fear of death as a result of repeated exposure and habituation). The theory states that while the desire for suicide is necessary, it is insufficient for an act of suicide to occur given that suicidal ideation is relatively common without leading to an actual suicide attempt. Thus, suicidal ideation must be accompanied by a capability for suicide. The ratio of self-harm behavior to deaths by suicide is approximately 20:1 in younger adults, whereas in older adults the ratio is approximately 4:1 [10]. This lower ratio of attempted to completed suicides in the older adults truly highlights the extreme lethality of suicidal behaviors in late life.

As applied to BPD, several key characteristics of this disorder may increase the desire and capability for suicide, including:

- repeated acts of self-harm or suicide attempts leading to pain habituation;
- fear of abandonment causing feelings of thwarted belongingness;
- feelings of self-hate and shame contributing to the perception of burdensomeness.

In older adults, the Interpersonal Theory of Suicide proposes that many factors may elevate the risk of late-life suicide [11]. More specifically, older adults who experience social isolation (e.g., living alone, loss of a spouse, loneliness) are at risk of thwarted belongingness, and those who require assistance with basic or instrumental activities of daily living, may increasingly perceive themselves as being a burden to others. While these factors may increase suicidal ideation, other factors may increase the capability for suicide, including the experience of chronic physical illness leading to repeated exposure and habituation to pain.

ASSESSMENT OF SUICIDAL RISK FACTORS

Although symptoms of BPD including impulsivity and self-harm behaviors tend to attenuate with age [7], suicide remains a significant clinical concern for older adults with BPD. A comprehensive suicide risk assessment identifies both risk and protective factors, and involves acquiring information through various sources including a review of the medical record, taking a history, interviewing family and friends when possible, and using risk assessment tools. Many countries have developed best practice guidelines for the screening and assessment of suicide in older adults, which includes the geriatric population with personality pathologies [12, 13].

Risk Factors: Individuals who have a history of prior suicidal behavior are at greater risk of dying by suicide. As recurrent suicidal behavior is a defining characteristic of BPD, the majority of patients will have at least one prior reported suicide attempt [14]. Attention must also be paid to the possibility of "passive" suicidal attempts amongst older adults, often referred to as "indirect self-destructive behaviors," which can include refusal to eat, take life-sustaining medications, or follow medical advice. Such self-injurious behaviors can serve as a way of communicating one's distress or an effort to hasten death. These self-destructive behaviors can be commonplace in long-term care settings. Interestingly, there has been little evidence of a relationship between depression and self-destructive behaviors [15]. Some proposed that self-injurious behaviors are due to poor impulse control and physical isolation [16]. The variation in the subtypes of self-injurious behaviors and methods chosen may be predicated on a number of factors, including psychosocial circumstances of living in a restricted residential treatment facility (and perhaps self-imposed isolation) versus living independently at home.

The presence of suicidal ideation and death ideation is another significant risk factor for suicide. However, older adults often under-report depressive and suicidal symptoms when compared with their younger counterparts [17], and thus it is important for clinicians to be vigilant in screening for suicidal risk factors even in the absence of overt suicidal ideation.

Other risk factors include comorbid psychiatric illness, in particular mood disorders and substance abuse, physical illness or the perception of physical illness, negative life events, and functional impairment [12]. Notably, BPD symptoms such as mood dysregulation, impulsivity, and aggression, are independent risk factors for suicide and self-harm behavior [1].

Protective Factors: Protective factors or resiliency of the patient may mitigate the risk of suicide. Several protective factors have been identified, including older adults who recognize the meaning and purpose of life, have active interests, have social contact with family and friends, exhibit better health care practices, and have moderate alcohol consumption [12].

Several standardized measurement tools have been created for use with older adults. We outline below examples of two such instruments:

- *Geriatric Suicide Ideation Scale* [18]. This is a 31-item self-report questionnaire with strong reliability and validity. The items tap active and passive thoughts about death and suicide, presence of a suicidal plan, value and meaning in life, and losses in the areas of physical functioning, social relationships, and status. One item taps previous suicidal behavior. Unlike many other tools, this questionnaire measures both suicide ideation and psychological resilience, and it contains four subscales (suicidal ideation, death ideation, loss of personal and social worth, and perceived meaning in life) which, according to the authors, can be used as stand-alone measures for risk assessment in cases where there is insufficient time to administer the full questionnaire.
- *Reasons for Living Scale – Older Adult Version* [19]. The focus of this measure is on resiliency factors, and scores tend to correlate negatively with measures of depression and suicidal ideation. The authors highlight the need to complement conventional suicide risk assessments, which tend to focus primarily on risk factors, with measures that assess for protective factors that may mitigate suicidal risk.

MANAGEMENT OF SUICIDE IN GERIATRIC BORDERLINE PERSONALITY DISORDER

Because patients with BPD frequently present with crises and chronic self-injurious behaviors and suicidal ideation, it is often challenging to accurately estimate suicidal risk, and to know which presentations merit increased monitoring. As previously discussed, risk assessment should include assessment of current mood symptoms, recent stressors and life events, comorbid substance misuse, and presence of available supports.

Figure 8-2 depicts strategies to minimize the risk of suicidal behaviors with special considerations for institutional settings [20-24]. For example, when assessing Mrs. B's potential for self-harm behavior, the focus should be on exploring:

- types of self-injury in which she engages (e.g., overdosing, and refusing meals, medical treatment, and personal care);
- onset and course of self-injurious behavior (e.g., longstanding and pervasive pattern);
- suicidal ideation during or before her self-injury (e.g., threats to harm herself);
- severity and impairment caused by self-injury (e.g., dehydration or other clinical syndromes in an already compromised physical state);
- possible functions served by her self-injury (e.g., attempt to communicate distress);
- intensity and frequency of self-injury behaviors (e.g., when perceived loneliness and fear of abandonment).

Residential Facility/Emergency Department Physician	*Inpatient Physician*
• Identify triggers for suicidal ideation/self-harm (stressors, losses, worsening physical health, change in housing/move to residential facility).	• Hospitalizations should be brief with the goal of stabilization and preparation for outpatient treatment.
• Are these triggers ongoing or time-limited?	• Set a mutually agreed upon discharge date with the patient early on.
• What has changed between the time of initial suicidality and the present to lower risk?	• Maintain clear and consistent patient-physician boundaries; these boundaries are themselves a therapeutic construct.
• If no change → consider admission.	• Use motivational interviewing to increase the patient's motivation for treatment.
• Treat the patient with empathy and respect; dismissive or antagonistic responses can provoke impulsive self-harm behaviors.	• Liaise with knowledgeable informants to obtain collateral history; i.e. nursing/assisted living facility staff, family members, outpatient therapist.
• The consultant physician faces a dilemma where discharge may be perceived as abandonment, and admission may lead to regression; awareness needed that both may increase suicidal risk.	• If possible, have a family meeting to discuss precipitants to the admission.
• If possible, convey this dilemma to the patient and involve them in the disposition decision-making process to encourage personal responsibility for one's safety.	• Treat comorbid psychiatric symptoms, but avoid excessive focus on illness and pharmacotherapy, as this may worsen regression by encouraging the patient to assume a passive sick role.
	• If possible avoid prescription of benzodiazepines, due to high potential for abuse, and the risk of worsening mood dysregulation in BPD patients, as well as risks of falls and cognitive impairment in the elderly.
	• BPD patients tend to provoke strong countertransference reactions in health care providers and to cause splitting amongst the health care team; educate team members about this common dynamic.

Figure 8-2. Strategies to Minimize Suicidality in Geriatric Borderline Patients in Institutional Settings [20-24].

It is important to identify Mrs. B's risk factors for self-injury and suicide (e.g., prior suicidal behavior, present suicidal ideation, physical illness, and functional impairment), as well as her protective factors (e.g., intact family and available social supports). A comprehensive risk assessment will guide clinical management by Mrs. B's health care team at the residential facility.

Although the mainstay for most patients with BPD will be a psychotherapeutic approach such as dialectical behavior therapy, medications are often used to alleviate symptoms such as mood dysregulation, impulsivity and aggression. As noted earlier, these symptoms are independent risk factors for suicide and self-harm [1], and thus require particular attention. For more detailed discussions on psychotherapy and pharmacotherapy modalities in BPD, please refer to Chapters 10 and 11, respectively.

It is important to note that several core features of BPD were unaffected by any of the medications studied, namely fears of abandonment, chronic feelings of emptiness, identity disturbance, and dissociation [25]. Lithium is frequently used to treat affective instability, despite a surprising lack of empirical support for its use in BPD. In a 2013 systematic review and meta-analysis, Cipriani et al. [26] concluded that lithium may be an effective treatment for reducing the risk of suicide in the mood disorder population, specifically in those with bipolar and unipolar mood disorders, although it was not found to be beneficial in reducing self-harm. Lithium likely exerts its antisuicidal effect by reducing the relapse of mood disorders, and by decreasing aggression and impulsivity [26]. Thus far, there is no evidence that lithium reduces suicidal risk in the BPD population. One controlled study on lithium in BPD carried out in by Links et al. in 1990 failed to demonstrate efficacy [27]. There are older studies supporting the use of lithium in personality disorders (although not BPD specifically), which focused on impulsivity and aggression rather than mood stability [28-30].

Pharmacotherapy with mood stabilizers and low-dose antipsychotics may be used as needed to target some of the key distressing symptoms of BPD. However, the current evidence does not suggest effectiveness for the overall severity of BPD, and medication should be used to augment psychotherapy.

KEY POINTS: SUICIDALITY IN GERIATRIC BORDERLINE PERSONALITY DISORDER: CLINICAL APPROACHES AND MANAGEMENT

- Geriatric patients with BPD are an especially high-risk group for suicide.
- There is an increasing need for prevention strategies to minimize the number of older lives tragically lost to suicide.
- Health care teams should be educated and trained in suicide risk assessment, treatment interventions and risk management practices.
- Health care providers must strive to remain empathic and consistent in our clinical management of this high-risk group.

REFERENCES

[1]   American Psychiatric Association: Practice guideline for the treatment of patients with borderline personality disorder. *Am J Psychiatry.* 2001; 158(10):1-52.

[2]   Centers for Disease Control and Prevention. Injury Prevention and Control: Data and Statistics (WISQARS). http://www.cdc.gov/injury/ wisqars/index.html. Accessed December 27, 2014.

[3]   Goodman M, Roiff T, Oakes AH, Paris J. Suicide risk and management in borderline personality disorder. *Curr Psychiatry Rep.* 2012; 14: 79-85.

[4]   Korzekwa MI, Dell PF, Links PS, Thabane L, Webb SP. Estimating the prevalence of borderline personality disorder in psychiatric outpatients using a two-phase procedure. *Compr Psychiatry.* 2008; 49(4):380-386.

[5]   American Psychiatric Association. Practice guideline for the assessment and treatment of patients with suicidal behavior. *Am J Psychiatry.* 2003; 160(11 Suppl): 1-60.

[6]   American Psychiatric Association. *Diagnostic and Statistical Manual of Mental Disorders* 5th ed. Arlington, VA: *American Psychiatric Publishing.* 2013: 646-649.

[7]   Morgan T, Chelminski I, Young D, Dalrymple K, Zimmerman M. Differences between older and younger adults with borderline personality disorder on clinical presentation and impairment. *J Psychiatr Res.* 2013; 47: 1507-1513.

[8]   Rosowsky E, Gurian B. Impact of borderline personality disorder in late life on systems of care. *Hosp Community Psychiatry.* 1992; 43(4): 386-389.

[9]   Van Orden K, Witte T, Cukrowicz K, Braithwaite S, Selby E, Joiner T. The Interpersonal theory of suicide. *Psychol Rev.* 2010; 117(2): 575-600.

[10] Conwell Y, Duberstein P, Cox C, Herrmann J, Forbes N, Caine E. Age differences in behaviors leading to completed suicide. *Am J Geriatr Psychiatry.* 1988; 6(2): 22-126.

[11] Van Orden K, Conwell Y. Suicides in late life. *Curr Psychiatry Rep.* 2012; 13(3): 234-241.

[12] Canadian Coalition for Seniors Mental Health (2006). *National Guidelines for Seniors Mental Health: The Assessment of Suicide Risk and Prevention of Suicide.* http://www.ccsmh.ca/en/natlguidelines/ suicide.cfm. Accessed September 17, 2014.

[13] Lapierre S, Erlangsen A, Waern M, et al. The International Research Group for Suicide among the Elderly. A systematic review of elderly suicide prevention programs. *Crisis.* 2011; 32(2): 88-98.

[14] Soloff P, Lis J, Kelly T, Cornelius J, Ulrich R. Risk factors for suicidal behavior in borderline personality disorder. *Am J Psychiatry.* 1994; 151: 1316-1323.

[15] Draper B, Brodaty H, Low LF, Richards V, Paton H, Lie D. Self-destructive behaviors in nursing home residents. *J Am Geriatr Soc.* 2002; 50(2): 354-358.

[16] Mahgoub N, Klimstra S, Kotbi N, Docherty JP. Self-injurious behavior in the nursing home setting. *Int J Geriatr Psychiatry.* 2011; 26(1): 27-30.

[17] Blazer D, Bachar J, Manton K. Suicide in late life: Review and commentary. *J Am Geriatr Soc.* 1986; 34(7): 519-525.

[18] Heisel M, Flett G. The development and initial validation of the geriatric suicide ideation scale. *Am J Geriatr Psychiatry.* 2006; 14: 742-751.

[19] Edelstein B, Heisel M, McKee D, et al. Development and psychometric evaluation of the Reasons for Living - Older Adults Scale: a suicide risk assessment inventory. *Gerontologist.* 2009; 49(6): 736–745.

[20] Gregory RJ. Managing Suicide Risk in Borderline Personality Disorder. *Psychiatric Times.* May 1, 2012. http://www.psychiatrictimes.com/ articles/managing-suicide-risk-borderline-personality-disorder/page/0/1. Accessed September 20, 2014.

[21] Cowdry RW, Gardner DL. Pharmacotherapy of borderline personality disorder. Alprazolam, carbamazepine, trifluoperazine, and tranylcypromine. *Arch Gen Psychiatry.* 1988; 45: 111-119.

[22] Main TF. The ailment. *Br J Med Psychol.* 1957; 30: 129-145.

[23] Linehan MM, Comtois KA, Murray AM, et al. Two-year randomized controlled trial and follow-up of dialectical behavior therapy versus therapy by experts for suicidal behaviors and borderline personality disorder. *Arch Gen Psychiatry.* 2006; 63: 757-766.

[24] Zanarini MC, Frankenburg FR, Fitzmaurice G. Defense Mechanisms Reported by Patients with Borderline Personality Disorder and Axis II Comparison Subjects Over 16 Years of Prospective Follow-Up: Description and Prediction of Recovery. *Am J Psychiatry.* 2013; 170: 111-120.

[25] Gelenberg AJ. Borderline Personality Disorder: A Role for Medication? *Biol Therapies in Psychiatry.* 2010; 33(5): http://www.btpnews.com/ article/2010/05/01/Borderline-Personality-Disorder-A-Role-for-Medication. Accessed September 28, 2014.

[26] Cipriani A, Hawton K, Stockton S, Geddes JR. Lithium in the prevention of suicide in mood disorders: updated systematic review and meta-analysis. *BMJ.* 2013; 346: f3646.

[27] Links P, Steiner M, Boiago I, Irwin D. Lithium therapy for borderline patients: preliminary findings. *J Personal Disord.* 1990; 4: 173–181.

[28] Sheard MH. Lithium in the treatment of aggression. *J Nerv Ment Dis.* 1975; 160: 108–118.

[29] Sheard MH, Marini JL, Bridges CI, Wagner E. The effect of lithium on impulsive aggressive behavior in man. *Am J Psychiatry.* 1976; 133: 1409–1413.

[30] Tupin JP, Smith DB, Clanon TL, Kim LI, Nugent A, Groupe A. The long-term use of lithium in aggressive prisoners. *Compr Psychiatry.* 1973; 14: 311–317.

In: Borderline Personality Disorder in Older Adults   ISBN: 978-1-63482-221-3
Editors: A. Hategan, J. A. Bourgeois, G. L. Xiong   © 2015 Nova Science Publishers, Inc.

Chapter 9

PSYCHIATRY AND THE LAW: PERSPECTIVES IN GERIATRIC BORDERLINE PERSONALITY DISORDER

Usha Parthasarathi[1,], MBBS, Yuri A. Alatishe[2], MD and Daniel L. Ambrosini[3], LLB/BCL, MSc, PhD*

[1]Associate Clinical Professor
Department of Psychiatry and Behavioural Neurosciences
McMaster University, Hamilton, ON, Canada
[2]Assistant Clinical Professor, Forensic Psychiatrist
St. Joseph's Healthcare Hamilton
Department of Psychiatry and Behavioural Neurosciences
McMaster University, Hamilton, ON, Canada
[3]Assistant Professor, Legal Counsel, Forensic Psychiatry Program,
St. Joseph's Healthcare Hamilton
Department of Psychiatry and Behavioural Neurosciences
McMaster University, Hamilton, ON, Canada

Clinicians are often called upon to assess mental capacity of older adults in contexts involving civil and criminal law. Assessing decisional capacity is an important, yet complex and individualized task that involves medical, legal, and ethical considerations. Cognitive and personality issues influence the nature and process of how individuals make decisions, and how clinicians conduct capacity assessments of older adults with borderline personality disorder (BPD). Using a clinical scenario, this chapter highlights some of the practices, safeguards, and obligations in assessing mental capacity, particularly in the context of forensic psychiatry, specific to older adults with BPD.

---

* Corresponding author: uparthas@stjoes.ca

INTRODUCTION

The need to assess whether someone is mentally capable can arise in several contexts in the civil setting (e.g., conservatorship, power of attorneys, wills, substitute decision-making) and in the criminal context (e.g., determining "right from wrong", fitness hearings, instruction to legal counsel) [1, 2]. Incompetency is a judicial determination, whereas incapacity indicates a functional inability as determined by a clinician [3]. The legal designation of "incompetent" is applied to a person who fails one of the mental tests of capacity, and the adjudication of "incompetence" by a court is subject or issue specific. The legal principles that apply when assessing decision-making capacity, with relevance to geriatric BPD, will be further detailed in this chapter. While formal capacity instruments are recommended to obtain an objective view of mental capacity, such as the MacArthur Competence Assessment Tool for Treatment [4] or the Capacity to Consent to Treatment Instrument [5], these instruments are not the only factor clinicians, judges, and lawyers will contemplate and it is often necessary to contextualize decisional capacity with the mental disorder in question [1, 6].

BPD has been viewed by some legal scholars with controversy, irrespective of how it may be understood by clinicians. One of the reasons for such skepticism is the higher level of scrutiny when comparing personality disorders with other clinical disorders such as schizophrenia where cognitive disorganization, delusions, and/or hallucinations may be present and impacting someone's ability to make rational decisions. However, transient, stress-related psychotic symptoms (usually paranoia) may also be present in BPD. Second, this chapter touches on older adults with BPD, which itself raises distinctive issues around decision-making for vulnerable persons experiencing cognitive decline. Therefore, there is an additional responsibility to be alert to and safeguard against potential biases of ageism when making capacity assessments with older persons [1, 7]. Third, this chapter focuses on institutional settings such as hospitals rather than on individuals living in the community, which presumes a higher level of supervision and monitoring if the person is a danger to themselves or others [8]. The following is a case description of an older adult with BPD to illustrate various clinical scenarios wherein assessment of decisional capacity may arise.

Case – Mr. J

Mr. J, a 70-year-old man, was brought to the hospital by the police for a psychiatric assessment. Mr. J's neighbor had called the police to report that Mr. J had made death threats to him and that he feared for his life. When police came to investigate, they found Mr. J in an agitated state shouting from his balcony, "I am a citizen. I have every right to be here…these people are trying to kill me! They are liars! I'm going to kill them!"

Mr. J was known to have chronic mental illnesses. He had been admitted to a psychiatric hospital three times in the last ten years, and had been diagnosed with a major depressive disorder, anxiety disorder, and BPD. Recently, he was diagnosed with an early stage of a major frontotemporal neurocognitive disorder. Mr. J's wife described him as a difficult, eccentric man who had longstanding anger issues. Police had been called for "domestic incidents" in the past. She was concerned about significant changes in his personality more recently. He had been more irritable, aggressive, and disinhibited and would frequently make sexual comments, use racial slurs, and utter death threats. Recently, he had been arguing with his neighbors over reports of noise nuisance. Subsequently, he started to ruminate that his neighbors were trying to kill him but would not give details, and he wanted to move from their residence to get away from "the scumbags." He had signed a lease for a new apartment a week ago and was also considering buying a gun for "self-defense." Mr. J's wife asked his clinical team:

"Can he be allowed to sign the lease? Can he buy a firearm?"

On clinical examination, Mr. J was oriented to place and time. He was acutely agitated and possibly psychotic, experiencing vague delusions of persecution. The psychiatrist recommended an inpatient admission and further evaluation. The psychiatry resident asked:

"Is the patient capable to consent for admission and treatment?"

During this admission, Mr. J's behavior fluctuated from day to day and there were no overt paranoid delusions reported any longer. His Montreal Cognitive Assessment score was 23 out of 30 and a brain magnetic resonance imaging showed bilateral focal frontal atrophy. Generally, he was able to have lucid conversations, but there were times when he struggled with his thoughts and speech. Hospital staff perceived his behavior on the unit as demanding and difficult. He made dramatic accusations to the staff such as, "You don't care about me, like others do." The staff also noted that when his wife visited him on the unit, he would be rude and argumentative towards her. Following one such visit, he declared that he was going to divorce his wife and marry a young patient he knew from another unit. He also told her that he was going to make a new will and bequest his estate to his "new love." He requested the social worker to help him find a new home when he got discharged. His nurse asked the psychiatrist:

"Does Mr. J have the capacity to make decisions related to marriage, divorce, and making a will?"
"Does Mr. J have the capacity to manage his finances?"
"Does Mr. J have the capacity to make his decisions regarding his living conditions?"

One day, Mr. J became extremely agitated during an altercation with Mr. X, a co-patient on the unit, and subsequently he expressed paranoid thoughts believing that Mr. X was disrespectful and talked about him behind his back with other patients. He hit Mr. X in the face that resulted in Mr. X losing three teeth. Mr. X filed a complaint to the police against Mr. J and he was arrested and charged with assault. During his initial appearance in court, Mr. J was not cooperative and the judge asked the lawyers:

"Is it your opinion that Mr. J even has the capacity or is fit to stand trial? Has a psychiatrist assessed whether he understands the nature of these legal proceedings?"

CIVIL ISSUES AND MENTAL CAPACITY

Legal issues related to performing capacity assessments of persons with BPD may arise in several settings including capacity to marry, to make a will, to enter a contract, to instruct legal counsel, and to accept or refuse medical treatment [9]. While most jurisdictions have legislation in place governing surrogate or substitute decision-making, the common law also applies on how capacity assessments are conducted by clinicians. There are legal and jurisdictional differences that also impact how and when capacity assessments may become necessary.

There are a few broad legal principles that apply across jurisdictions when assessing decision-making capacity. There is a rebuttable presumption that individuals with a mental disorder are mentally capable to make decisions autonomously. When a clinician is concerned by a patient's behavior, speech, and appearance that they may be incapable to understand or appreciate the information, a formal assessment should be undertaken to examine the patient's decisional capacity [6, 8]. Broadly speaking, clinicians should be aware that the legal test for mental capacity is rarely whether someone will make a wise decision or not, but often relates to the person having the ability to *understand* and *appreciate* the relevant information, and whether the individual is able to communicate their choices rationally [1, 6]. This means that while an individual with BPD may have capacity for some types of decisions, they may not have it for others such that mental capacity can vary across time and context.

BPD raises unique challenges in terms of assessing decision-making capacity. Various personality disorders can affect an individual's degree of mental capacity differently, and these disorders are also perceived differently by others, each with their own implicit biases. How different individuals present with BPD, with its various stages and types, have led some U.S. courts to rule that BPD does not constitute a mental disease or defect for the purpose of a competency determination [10, 11].

Whereas few would argue, for example, that paranoid personality disorder affects a person's ability to think rationally, or that histrionic personality disorder causes emotional overreaction, BPD tends to cause *both* emotional overreaction and thought disturbance. Persons with BPD have difficulty understanding how the reactions of others affect them and are often prone to rapid vacillations of emotional instability [10]. It is equally important for clinicians to determine the level of support family and friends can provide when decisions need to be made for persons with BPD given the interpersonal difficulties that often arise [1, 2].

BPD is characterized by a chaotic lifestyle, difficulty with relationships, tendencies to act in a manipulative manner, and self-injurious or suicidal acts [10]. As a result, those with BPD tend to underperform in terms of attention, cognitive flexibility, planning, and processing speed. They are typically impulsive and suffer from impaired volition in terms of their decisions [10]. Still, there is a high degree of heterogeneity in terms of how any single individual will meet the current diagnostic criteria for BPD, which makes performing capacity assessments difficult. Clinicians should evaluate a person's authentic preferences, beliefs, and values over time to determine whether their legal declarations are an accurate representation of their wishes [1]. The emotional lability, changeability, and actions without consideration of consequences make performing capacity assessments challenging [10]. With frequent splitting, it can become difficult for clinicians to evaluate a person's authentic identity to determine if those wishes represent one's long-term goals. This becomes an important factor when individuals with BPD want to complete a will or a power of attorney, for example [9, 10, 12]. Similarly, a pervasive pattern of unstable relationships and conflict with others means that clinicians will need to be alert to changes in a surrogate or substitute decision-maker [10, 13].

Legal issues associated with BPD also arise in the family law context where relationships may break down and family, clinicians, and lawyers find themselves dealing with highly irrational and impulsive decisions [13]. This can arise with end-of-life decisions, parental capacity assessments, or changes to wills or powers of attorneys [14, 15]. Situations may occur when it is prudent to postpone important legal decisions until someone with BPD has become less emotionally labile and has returned to what is the closest version of their true self. The changeability factor requires psychiatrists to find the optimal time to discuss with patients, along with their family members, when and how to make critical decisions [1, 6, 15, 16]. This can be difficult if persons with BPD are having interpersonal challenges to the point of mistreating their own family members, clinicians, and lawyers who are trying to facilitate decisions [13, 16].

CRIMINAL ISSUES AND MENTAL CAPACITY

The aggressive behavior associated with BPD has puzzled clinicians and researchers, similar to other high risk personality disorders, and there often appears to be some degree of insight and empathy exhibited [17]. As a result, when criminal responsibility is an issue some wonder if persons with BPD should be held more or less responsible than those with other personality disorders. How volitional was the persons' action and to what extent does suffering from BPD diminish moral and legal responsibility in comparison to other personality disorders? Some suggest that persons with BPD actually have stable volitions, which allows for an easier assessment of the persons' character and authenticity of expressed wishes [18]. However, as older adults with BPD are more likely to suffer from general medical and cognitive issues (and also take multiple medications), the overall assessment of aggressive behavior in older adults with BPD is even more complex, as in Mr. J's case.

When an individual enters the forensic psychiatry system there are several domains of capacity encountered that are specific to psychiatry and the law. Fitness to stand trial and criminal responsibility are the most common type of assessments performed by a forensic psychiatrist. It should be noted that even when assessing an individual's capacity in the context of a fitness assessment the person is presumed to be capable until proven otherwise, usually on a balance of probabilities [18-20].

Every individual has the right to a fair trial when they have been charged with an offence. A fair trial is only possible if the accused has the capacity to understand the object and nature of the proceedings, the possible consequences of the proceedings and is able to communicate with counsel regarding how their defense is conducted. If there is concern that an accused's mental state is affecting their ability to meet these requirements the court will order that the accused be assessed by a psychiatrist to determine if he or she is "fit to stand trial" [19-21].

Case – Mr. J (Continued)

Mr. J. was not cooperative with his counsel during the initial proceedings and did not appear to understand fully; therefore, his competency to stand trial was brought into question by the judge. On psychiatric examination, Mr. J was found to be experiencing delusions and was subsequently suspicious and guarded in his behaviors. Despite his acute psychotic symptoms, Mr. J was able to demonstrate an understanding of why he was being charged, the legal situation he now found himself in, and the potential legal consequences. His unwillingness to cooperate with counsel was thought to be volitional (not a product of mental illness), and therefore not indicative of his incapacity to proceed with the legal process. Based on the clinical findings of the forensic psychiatrist, the legal decision-maker, in this case the judge, found that Mr. J did in fact have sufficient capacity to be found fit to stand trial and consequently allowed the trial to proceed.

Mr. J and his counsel put forth the defense that Mr. J was not guilty by reason of insanity when he committed the assault of the co-patient. A forensic psychiatric assessment was ordered by the court. The forensic psychiatrist was of the opinion that Mr. J was not suffering from a persistent psychotic process at the time of the offense. The patient, however, was emotionally disturbed and experienced acute paranoia that others were trying to hurt him. The forensic psychiatrist was of the opinion that the psychiatric symptoms were of such intensity that they rendered Mr. J incapable of appreciating the nature of his actions and their potential consequences. There was also evidence of a major frontotemporal neurocognitive disorder from clinical and neuroimaging examination that suggested the patient's executive function and judgment were impaired. The judge allowed the psychiatrist's opinion and testimony and the jury found Mr. J not guilty.

An assessment of criminal responsibility is essentially a determination of whether the accused had the mental capacity to form a criminal intent at the time the offence was committed [22]. For an individual to be found culpable of an offence he or she must have the criminal intent, commonly referred to as *mens rea* [22]. Therefore, when a psychiatrist assesses whether an accused may qualify for an insanity defense he must determine if the accused, at the time of the offence, was capable of appreciating the nature and quality of their actions and if he knew these actions were morally wrong. If an accused is found not guilty or not criminally responsible due to a mental disorder, he is often committed to a psychiatric facility for an indeterminate period to receive the necessary medical treatment while ensuring public safety. Diminished capacity, a related but distinct defense, is a determination that the accused should not be held fully criminally liable for their offense, as their mental capacity was diminished or impaired by mitigating factors (e.g., disease of the mind, brain injury, or intoxication) [23]. A defense of diminished capacity will not completely exonerate a person from criminal responsibility, but may serve to reduce the level of the offense and the applicable penalty [23, 24].

It is important to note that it is the accused's mental state at the *current* time that is critical to an assessment of fitness to stand trial, whereas it is the mental state at the *time of the offence* that is critical during an assessment of criminal responsibility (not guilty by reason of insanity). Although a mental illness/disease of the mind is necessary for an individual to be found incapable to stand trial or not guilty by reason of insanity, it is not sufficient.

KEY POINTS: PSYCHIATRY AND THE LAW: PERSPECTIVES IN GERIATRIC BORDERLINE PERSONALITY DISORDER

- The legal test for capacity varies across jurisdictions but often involves whether a person has the ability to *understand* and *appreciate* the relevant information and can communicate their choices rationally.
- Capacity assessments may be sought in various contexts for older adults with BPD.
- Older adults with BPD present unique challenges to conduct formal capacity assessments and a thoughtful systematic approach is necessary.

REFERENCES

[1]   Moye J, Marson DC, Edelstein B. Assessment of capacity in an aging society. *Am Psychol.* 2013; 68(3): 158-171.
[2]   Samsi K, Manthorpe J. Everyday decision-making in dementia: findings from a longitudinal interview study of people with dementia and family carers. *Int Psychogeriatr.* 2013; 25(6): 949-961.
[3]   Berg JW, Appelbaum PS, Grisso T. Constructing competence: Formulating standards of legal competence to make medical decisions. *Rutgers Law Rev.* 1996; 48(2): 345-371.
[4]   Appelbaum PS, Grisso T. The MacArthur Treatment Competence Study. I: Mental illness and competence to consent to treatment. *Law Hum Behav.* 1995; 19(2): 105-126.
[5]   Marson DC, Ingram KK, Cody HA, Harrell LE. Assessing the competency of patients with Alzheimer's disease under different legal standards. A prototype instrument. *Arch Neurol.* 1995; 52(10): 949-954.
[6]   Appelbaum PS, Grisso T. Assessing patients' capacities to consent to treatment. *N Engl J Med.* 1988; 319(25): 1635-1638.
[7]   Doron I. Mental incapacity, guardianship, and the elderly: an exploratory study of Ontariomer's disease under differend. *Can J Law Soc.* 2003; 18(1): 131-148.
[8]   Owen GS, Szmukler G, Richardson G, et al. Decision-making capacity for treatment in psychiatric and medical in-patients: cross-sectional, comparative study. *Br J Psychiatry.* 2013; 203(6): 461-467.
[9]   Sisti DA, Caplan AL. Accommodation without exculpation? The ethical and legal paradoxes of borderline personality disorder. *J Psychiatry Law.* 2012; 40: 75-92.
[10] American Psychiatric Association. *Diagnostic and Statistical Manual of Mental Disorders.* 5th ed. Washington, DC: American Psychiatric Publishing; 2013.
[11] Behnke SH, Saks ER. Therapeutic jurisprudence: informed consent as a clinical indication for the chronically suicidal patient with borderline personality disorder. *Loyola Los Angeles Law Review.* 1998; 31: 945-982.
[12] Roof JG. Testamentary capacity and guardianship assessments. *Psychiatr Clin North Am.* 2012; 35(4): 915-927.
[13] Crump D, Anderson JS. Effects upon divorce proceedings when a spouse suffers from Borderline Personality Disorder. *Family Law Quarterly.* 2009; 43(3); 571-586.
[14] Widera E, Steenpass V, Marson D, Sudore R. Finances in the older patient with cognitive impairment: "He didn't want me to take over". *JAMA.* 2011; 305(7): 698-706.

[15] Moberg PJ, Rick JH. Decision-making capacity and competency in the elderly: a clinical and neuropsychological perspective. *NeuroRehabilitation.* 2008; 23(5): 403-413.

[16] Margulies S. Representing the client from hell: divorce and the borderline client. *J Psychiatry Law.* 1997; 25: 347-363.

[17] Daffern M, Howells K. Aggressive behavior in high-risk personality disordered inpatients during prison and following admission to hospital. *Psychiatr Psychol Law.* 2007; 14(1): 26-34.

[18] Bonnie R. The competence of criminal defendants: A theoretical reformulation. *Behav Sci Law.* 1992; 10: 291-316.

[19] Alvaro LC. Competency: general principles and applicability in dementia. *Neurologia.* 2012; 27(5): 290-300.

[20] Otto RK. Competency to stand trial. *Appl Psychol Crim Justice.* 2006; 2(3): 82-113.

[21] Wulach JS. The incompetency plea: Abuses and reforms. *J Psychiatry Law.* 1980; 8:317-328.

[22] Dalby JT. The case of Daniel McNaughton: let's get the story straight. *Am J Forensic Psychiatry.* 2006; 27: 17-32.

[23] Felthous AR. Diminished capacity: Subterfuge or just defense? *AAPL Newsletter. J Am Acad Psychiatry Law.* 2000; 24(1): 10-11.

[24] Ogloff JRP. A comparison of insanity defense standards on juror decision making. *Law Hum Behav.* 1991; 15(5): 509-531.

In: Borderline Personality Disorder in Older Adults
Editors: A. Hategan, J. A. Bourgeois, G. L. Xiong

ISBN: 978-1-63482-221-3
© 2015 Nova Science Publishers, Inc.

Chapter 10

PSYCHOTHERAPY

Laura E. Kenkel[1,], MD and Andreea L. Seritan[2], MD*
[1]Associate Physician Diplomate
Health Sciences Assistant Clinical Professor
University of California, Davis
Department of Psychiatry and Behavioral Sciences
Sacramento, CA, US
[2]Associate Professor of Clinical Psychiatry
University of California, Davis
Department of Psychiatry and Behavioral Sciences
Sacramento, CA, US

Several psychotherapeutic modalities used in the treatment of patients with borderline personality disorder (BPD) are examined, with a focus on use in older adults in institutional settings. Supportive therapy requires a warm and involved therapist, and seeks to utilize a patient's existing strengths and resources. Dialectical behavior therapy (DBT) is a manualized approach combining elements of cognitive behavioral therapy and mindfulness that employs both individual therapy and group sessions to specifically treat patients with BPD. Transference focused psychotherapy is another manualized, individual therapy that makes use of transference interpretations, in an attempt to integrate the patient's fragmented internal object relations. Systems Training for Emotional Predictability and Problem Solving (STEPPS) is a manualized group program that educates patients on cognitive behavioral therapy principles, while also providing education to those in their support system. Nidotherapy emphasizes making environmental changes that minimize the effect of mental illness on the patient, rather than seeking to change the patient herself. Family therapy is an opportunity to examine the dynamics between patients and their family members. Most of these modalities can be utilized in institutional settings, and benefit from using a team approach.

---

* Corresponding author: Laura.kenkel@ucdmc.ucdavis.edu

Introduction

The range of psychotherapeutic interventions for BPD has grown over the last few decades [1]. Several psychotherapeutic modalities have been shown in randomized controlled trials to be effective for patients with BPD: DBT, mentalization based therapy, transference focused psychotherapy, schema focused therapy, STEPPS, and dynamic deconstructive therapy [2].

Evidence also supports the pharmacological management of affective dysregulation, impulsive behavioral dyscontrol, and cognitive perceptual symptoms, in combination with psychotherapy [3] (Also see Chapter 11). While some studies have focused on the clinical presentation of BPD in older adults [4, 5], less work has been done to examine the indications and utility of specific BPD focused therapies in this age group. Generally, only low numbers of geriatric patients are enrolled in randomized controlled studies, and research on the effectiveness of psychotherapeutic modalities is still emerging. Additionally, while there have been studies pertaining to the application of certain therapies to inpatient psychiatric units, not all the above therapies have been used or studied in institutional settings other than psychiatric facilities.

In this chapter, we will briefly review supportive therapy, DBT, transference focused therapy, STEPPS, and family therapy and their applications to older patients with BPD in institutional settings. Additionally, we will discuss nidotherapy, a unique therapeutic approach that provides an alternative way to treat those patients with BPD (as well as patients with other severe personality disorders) who seem intractable to other treatments [6].

1. Supportive Therapy

Supportive therapy, also known as client centered therapy, non-directive supportive therapy, or person centered therapy [7], is the most frequently utilized psychotherapy across all settings, which can be delivered in either individual or group format. Supportive therapy focuses on changing the patient's behavior by encouraging positive adaptive behaviors and a more effective utilization of environmental resources [8].

The therapist conducting supportive therapy is respectful and warm to the patient, empathizes and validates emotions, builds the patients' self-esteem and highlights their strengths [7]. Supportive therapy has a less well defined framework compared to other therapies, does not utilize transference interpretation and does not seek to actually change the patient's personality [8].

A supportive approach is indicated in the initial treatment of patients with BPD, until a solid therapeutic alliance is forged [9] (Also see Chapter 7), as well as in those hospitalized for acute medical or surgical illnesses. A variety of brief psychotherapeutic modalities can be utilized in medical settings, including elements of dynamic therapy, cognitive behavioral therapy or DBT [10].

A recent study comparing intensive mentalization based therapy (a combination of individual and group sessions) and biweekly group supportive therapy in patients with BPD found significant changes in both treatment groups on self-reported measures of general functioning, depression, and social functioning, and the number of BPD diagnostic criteria [11].

In his recent paper, Clark offers suggestions as to how supportive therapy can be integrated into case management for older adults with BPD, in settings ranging from nursing homes to intensive outreach programs [12]. For example, a social worker called to consult on a patient who is verbally abusive and severely disrupting the milieu of a nursing home unit, can utilize empathy and validation of feelings to build a therapeutic relationship with the patient, assess the patient's needs, and then facilitate communication between the patient and the primary team [12].

Case – Mrs. P

Mrs. P was a 67-year-old woman with schizoaffective disorder, BPD and history of alcohol, cocaine and opioid use, in remission. She also had multiple medical problems including obesity, diabetes mellitus type II, hepatitis C (secondary to intravenous drug use) and hypertension.

Mrs. P was divorced and had two children and two grandchildren. She was estranged from her son, who lived out of state; however she visited her daughter and babysat her granddaughters occasionally. Mrs. P was hospitalized for the surgical excision of a large benign abdominal tumor.

During her post-operative course, she refused to follow the nurses' recommendations to get out of bed and walk and took her medications inconsistently. A psychiatric consult was called. Mrs. P spent much of the time in the interview complaining about the poor care she felt she had been receiving from the inpatient team. The psychiatrist, Dr. A, listened empathically and then explored the patient's reasons for her poor adherence to treatment recommendations. Mrs. P stated that she felt the nurses and physicians only wanted her to become more independent so she could be discharged soon, whereas she thought she needed a lot more care at this time. Upon further inquiry, Mrs. P shared that, as a child, she had been neglected by her drug using mother, who would leave her and her siblings unattended for days, without food. Mrs. P recalled how she and her siblings used to make "mud cakes", dry them in the sun, and eat them. Dr. A interpreted that perhaps Mrs. P felt she would be abandoned by her medical team, the same way as her mother had done when she was a child. Mrs. P started crying and admitted that she felt no one loved her. After this session, Mrs. P started participating in her recovery. One week later, she was discharged to a nursing home facility.

2. DIALECTICAL BEHAVIOR THERAPY (DBT)

DBT is a manualized therapy, originally developed to treat patients with BPD, with an emphasis on those at high risk of suicide [13]. DBT combines cognitive behavioral therapy elements with mindfulness skills and consists of individual therapy sessions, group skills training sessions, skills generalization (usually accomplished through telephone calls between therapist and patient outside of the therapy hour) and a consultation team that supports the DBT therapists [13].

DBT is conducted in four stages: first, treating behavioral dysfunction, focusing on the most dangerous and/or disabling behaviors; second, assisting patients in experiencing emotions; third, focusing on dealing with other life stressors; and fourth, helping patients learn to experience joy and freedom [13]. A randomized, controlled trial comparing 1 year of DBT treatment to community treatment by experts (CTBE) for suicidal patients and patients with BPD, found that DBT was superior to CTBE in preventing suicide attempts, reducing emergency department visits and psychiatric hospitalizations for suicidal ideation [14].

The DBT manual has been adapted to make it more applicable for older adults with personality disorders by emphasizing techniques to address the greater despair and rigidity of older adults with BPD and including efforts to encourage openness to new experiences, strategies to deal with life stressors, and a module that compares looking forward (focusing on goals and planning) with looking back (development of a positive personal narrative, focus on forgiveness of others and self) [15].

Outpatient DBT manuals have also been modified for inpatient use, but there is no standard inpatient DBT manual that has been systematically tested [16]. Regardless of the therapeutic modality utilized in the inpatient setting, maintaining strict boundaries and closely monitoring countertransference feelings are crucial principles that will help manage splitting and projective identification phenomena [2, 17].

Case – Mrs. P (Continued)

One year later, Mrs. P had an argument with her daughter over parenting styles. She felt her daughter was too strict in reinforcing her children's bedtime and called Child Protective Services to report this alleged abuse. Her daughter was enraged, brought up the fact that Mrs. P had been physically abusive to her children during her 10 years of drug use, and completely severed ties with her. Mrs. P became despondent, paranoid (was convinced that her neighbors were spying on her at night), and attempted suicide by overdosing on her medications. She was admitted to a psychiatric unit, where she started participating in DBT groups.

The group therapist, Dr. B, first addressed the patients' suicidal ideation and self-harm impulses. Mrs. P's acute suicidal ideation resolved. She felt that finally, someone understood her suffering. She sought out Dr. B, asking to speak with her in private, and was dismissive to the psychiatric resident, Dr. C. She told Dr. C: "You are way too young, I can tell you don't know what you are doing", and "Dr. B is the only one who 'gets' me, she has a lot of experience". In staff meetings, Dr. C expressed his frustration with Mrs. P's demeaning attitude. Dr. B educated the team on splitting and common countertransference pitfalls in treating patients with BPD. The team agreed on a treatment plan and consistently reinforced it, setting limits regarding Mrs. P's behavior. Mrs. P was discharged home with the recommendation to attend a partial hospital program, consisting of DBT and medication management groups. Over the next 4 weeks, Mrs. P learned basic mindfulness skills, which allowed her to better tolerate her emotions.

3. TRANSFERENCE FOCUSED PSYCHOTHERAPY

Transference focused psychotherapy is another manualized therapy for patients with BPD, based on a model of contemporary psychoanalytic object relations theory [18, 19]. Transference focused psychotherapy utilizes modified techniques suited to patients with severe personality disorders who may not respond well to typical psychoanalytic approaches [20]. Transference focused psychotherapy approaches patients with BPD as suffering from identity diffusion, which is an inability to assimilate the concepts of self and others [18]. Transference interpretations are carefully titrated, with the goal of integrating the patient's fragmented internal object relations [18]. Transference focused psychotherapy is conducted in individual sessions, two to three times per week [18].

The transference focused psychotherapist first establishes a therapeutic frame by means of a treatment contract that provides a safe space for patient expression [21]. The therapist then in a noncritical and nonjudgmental way uses clarification, confrontation and interpretation to explore the objection relations that are the basis of the patient's affect, actions and interactions [21].

These techniques promote increased reflection, leading toward better integration of fragmented object relations, which further leads to improved control of affect and continued improvement in ability to reflect and contextualize [21]. Transference focused psychotherapy also utilizes countertransference to inform the therapist's understanding of the patient's internal experience, aspects from which the patient may be split off [19]. The primary contraindications for transference focused psychotherapy are patients with clear antisocial personality disorder, patients with narcissistic personality disorder with severe antisocial features, or other patients who have a history of chronic dishonesty, which would significantly impair communication in the therapy [18].

4. SYSTEMS TRAINING FOR EMOTIONAL PREDICTABILITY AND PROBLEM SOLVING (STEPPS)

STEPPS is a manualized psychoeducational program based on cognitive behavioral therapy principles, developed for patients with BPD [22]. It is relatively brief, with twenty 2-hour long weekly sessions which are structured similarly to seminars [23]. STEPPS is notably different from other BPD focused therapies, in that it is solely conducted in groups, and has no individual psychotherapy component [1], although it is designed to be added to an existing regimen of individual therapy outside of the STEPPS program [22]. STEPPS was designed to make use of the patient's support system (both social and professional), by providing education to their family and/or other identified support system members, and by teaching patients to more effectively use their support system [22]. There are three stages in the STEPPS training: 1) educating patients on BPD as a disorder, and the ability to manage it by learning appropriate behavioral and emotional skills; 2) teaching skills to manage the cognitive and emotional aspects of BPD; and 3) teaching skills to manage the behavioral aspects of BPD [22]. Figure 10-1 summarizes the STEPPS training stages [22, 23].

Step 1: Psychoeducation

    a. Recognition of BPD as a disorder with a specific
       treatment and hopeful prognosis

Step 2: Cognitive and emotional skills training

    a. Distancing

    b. Communication

    c. Challenging thoughts

    d. Distracting

    e. Problem management

Step 3: Behavior skills training

    a. Goal setting

    b. Healthy eating and sleep hygiene

    c. Exercise and physical health

    d. Relaxation and leisure behaviors

    e. Health monitoring

    f. Avoiding abusive behaviors

    g. Interpersonal effectiveness

Figure 10-1. STEPPS training stages (adapted from 22, 23).

5. NIDOTHERAPY

Nidotherapy, or nest therapy (after the Latin word *nidus*), is a treatment that emphasizes collaboration between therapist and patient, and aims to modify the patient's environment to help diminish the effect of a mental illness on both the individual suffering from the illness, and the society that the individual exists within [24]. Nidotherapy focuses on changing the patient's environment and may be applied to patients with chronic mood and psychotic disorders particularly resistant to treatment, as well as personality disorders [6, 24]. Interventions range from relatively simple, for example installing an additional deadbolt to the door for a patient who feels unsafe or paranoid, to more complex, such as managing the patient's money so they can purchase higher quality furnishings, to help them feel more comfortable inviting friends or family to visit [25].

Nidotherapy is also notably different from other approaches in that progress is measured via mutually agreed upon environmental targets and functional gain, rather than change in the patient [6]. The nidotherapist works separately from other clinical team members, so as to be an independent treatment advocate for the patient [26]. This provides potential advantages in that the nidotherapist can act as a professional advocate for the patient, and provide new perspectives to the clinical team regarding their relationship with the patient, but also has some disadvantages, particularly if the clinical team does not have sufficient education about nidotherapy, or if there is a lack of communication between the nidotherapist and the clinical team [26]. In a recent study of nidotherapy applied in assertive community outreach programs, patients who received an average of 20 hours of nidotherapy over a year had less hospital admissions [27]. Nidotherapy is primarily an outpatient modality and its utility may be limited in institutional settings due to challenges such as staff changes and facility policies [26].

6. FAMILY THERAPY

Family involvement in the treatment of older patients with BPD is important, although it may be complicated by long-standing conflicts between patients and their adult children. Therapists need to help the children place their parents into a more age-appropriate context and to understand the patients' limitations due to physical or mental illness [17]. A useful strategy is to review communication scenarios between patients and their family members and make suggestions for alternative responses or other behavioral changes [17].

In summary, Table 10-1 illustrates the psychotherapies for patients with BPD that may be used in inpatient settings [7, 8, 15, 17, 19, 22, 25].

Table 10-1. Psychotherapies for patients with BPD that may be used in inpatient settings

Psychotherapy	Structure	Frequency	Duration	Manualized	May be used in inpatient settings	Therapeutic goals
Supportive therapy [7, 8]	Individual +/- group	Flexible	Flexible	No	Yes	Emphasize patient strengths and support systems
Dialectical behavior therapy [15]	Individual + group	Weekly individual Weekly group	Outpatient: ≥ 6 months Inpatient: ≥ 2 months	Yes	Yes	Develop CBT and mindfulness skills
Transference focused psychotherapy [19]	Individual	Twice a week	≥ 1 year	Yes	No	Integrate internal object relations via transference interpretation
STEPPS [22]	Group	Weekly, 2-hour sessions	20 weeks	Yes	Possibly, with modifications	Psychoeducation, CBT principles
Nidotherapy [25]	Individual	Flexible	Flexible (usually 10 sessions)	No	Possibly, with modifications	Change the environment to better meet the patient's needs
Family therapy [17]	Family	Flexible	Flexible	No	Yes	Improve family dynamics and functioning

Note: BPD, Borderline Personality Disorder; CBT, Cognitive Behavioral Therapy; STEPPS, Systems Training for Emotional Predictability and Problem Solving.

Case – Mrs. P (Continued)

Six months later, Mrs. P completed the partial hospital program and was referred to Dr. D, an outpatient psychiatrist. Dr. D offered supportive therapy and medication management. One day, Mrs. P slipped and fell in her apartment and broke her left femur, which led to a lengthy hospitalization. She was discharged to a nursing home facility. At the end of Mrs. P's stay at the nursing home, the social worker and nursing team determined that she would not be able to live independently because she was not managing her medications adequately and due to her high risk of falls. Despite the team's efforts to engage Mrs. P's daughter, her family remained estranged. Mrs. P went to live in an assisted living facility, where Dr. D continued to follow her with monthly home visits.

KEY POINTS: PSYCHOTHERAPY

- A team approach is often necessary in order to achieve best outcomes in the treatment of individuals with BPD, as is the clear delineation of boundaries.
- Several psychotherapeutic modalities have good evidence in the treatment of patients with BPD, although limited data exist for older individuals with BPD.
- Cognitive behavioral therapy, DBT, STEPPS and supportive therapy can be used in institutional settings including medical facilities, partial hospital programs, and psychiatric inpatient units.
- Mental health care providers should be familiar with elements of all these therapies and be able to modify and apply them as dictated by patient needs.
- Combining psychotherapy with medication management has been proven to be effective in the treatment of patients with BPD, including in the older population.

REFERENCES

[1]   Stoffers JM, Völlm BA, Rücker G, Timmer A, Huband N, Lieb K. Psychological therapies for people with borderline personality disorder (Review). *Cochrane Database Syst Rev.* 2012; 8:CD005652.

[2]   Gabbard GO. Cluster B personality disorders: Borderline. In: *Psychodynamic Psychiatry in Clinical Practice* 5th ed. Arlington, VA: American Psychiatric Publishing, Inc.; 2014: 444-470.

[3]   American Psychiatric Association. Treatment recommendations for patients with borderline personality disorder. In: *Practice Guidelines for the Treatment of Psychiatric Disorders.* Arlington, VA: American Psychiatric Publishing, Inc.; 2004: 770-776.

[4]   Arens EA, Stopsack M, Spitzer C, et al. Borderline personality disorder in four different age groups: a cross-sectional study of community residents in Germany. *J Pers Disord.* 2013; 27: 196-207.

[5]   Morgan TA, Chelminski I, Young D, Dalrymple K, Zimmerman M. Differences between older and younger adults with borderline personality disorder on clinical presentation and impairment. *J Psychiatry Res.* 2013; 47: 1507-1513.

[6]   Tyrer P. Nidotherapy: A new approach to the treatment of personality disorder. *Acta Psychiatr Scand.* 2002; 105: 469-472.

[7]   Jacobs N, Reupert A. The effectiveness of supportive counselling, based on Rogerian principles: a systematic review of recent international and Australian research. *Psychotherapy and Counselling Federation of Australia.* 2014. http://www.pacfa.org.au/wp-content/uploads/2012/10/PACFA-Supportive-Counselling-literature-review-May-2014-Final.pdf

[8]   Conte HR. Review of research in supportive psychotherapy: An Update. *Am J Psychother.* 1994; 48 (4): 494-504.

[9]   Gabbard GO, Seritan AL, Allison SE. Psychodynamic treatment. In: Simon RI, Hales RE, eds. *Textbook of Suicide Risk Assessment and Management* 2nd ed. Arlington, VA: American Psychiatric Publishing, Inc.; 2012: 251-262.

[10]   Lipsitt DR. Psychotherapy. In: Wise MG, Rundell JR, eds. *Textbook of Consultation-Liaison Psychiatry.* 2nd ed. Washington, DC: American Psychiatric Publishing, Inc.; 2002: 1027-1051.

[11]   Jørgensen CR, Freund C, Bøye R, Jordet H, Andersen D, Kjølbye M. Outcome of mentalization-based and supportive psychotherapy in patients with borderline personality disorder: a randomized trial. *Acta Psychiatr Scand.* 2013; 127: 305-317.

[12]   Clark S. Integration of supportive psychotherapy with case management for older adults with borderline personality disorder. *J Gerontol Soc Work.* 2011; 54(6): 627-638.

[13]   Lynch TR, Trost WT, Salsman N, Linehan MM. Dialectical behavior therapy for borderline personality disorder. *Annu Rev Clin Psychol.* 2007; 3: 181-205.

[14]   Linehan MM, Comtois KA, Murray AM, Brown MZ, Gallop RJ, Heard HL, Korslund KE, Tutek DA, Reynolds SK, Lindenboim N. Two-year randomized controlled trial and follow-up of dialectical behavior therapy vs therapy by experts for suicidal behaviors and borderline personality disorder. *Arch Gen Psychiatry.* 2006; 63(7):757-766.

[15]   Lynch TR, Cheavens JS, Cukrowicz KC, Thorp SR, Bronner L, Beyer J. Treatment of older adults with co-morbid personality disorder and depression: a dialectical behavior therapy approach. *Int J Geriatr Psychiatry* 2007; 22: 131-143.

[16]   Bloom JM, Woodward EN, Susmaras T, Pantalone DW. Use of dialectical behavior therapy in inpatient treatment of borderline personality disorder: a systematic review. *Psychiatr Serv.* 2012; 63(9): 881-888.

[17]   Abrams RC, Sadavoy J. Personality disorders. In: Sadavoy J, Jarvik LF, Grossberg GT, Meyers BS, eds. *Comprehensive Textbook of Geriatric Psychiatry* 3rd ed. New York, NY: Norton; 2004; 701-721.

[18]   Kernberg OF, Yeomans FE, Clarkin JF, Levy KN. Transference focused therapy: overview and update. *Int J Psychoanal* 2008; 89: 601-620.

[19]   Yeomans FE, Levy KN, Caligor E. Transference-focused psychotherapy. *Psychotherapy (Chic).* 2013; 50(3): 449-453.

[20]   Caligor E, Diamond D, Yeomans FE, Kernberg OF. The interpretive process in the psychoanalytic psychotherapy of borderline personality pathology. *J Am Psychoanal Assoc.* 2009; 57: 271-301.

[21]   Levy KN, Clarkin JF, Yeomans FE, Scott LN, Wasserman RH, Kernberg OF. The mechanisms of change in the treatment of borderline personality disorder with transference focused psychotherapy. *J Clin Psychol.* 2006; 62(4): 481-501.

[22] Blum N, Pfohl B, St. John D, Monahan P, Black DW. STEPPS: A cognitive-behavioral systems-based group treatment for outpatients with borderline personality disorder – a preliminary report. *Compr Psychiatry.* 2002; 43: 301-310.

[23] Blum N, St. John D, Pfohl B, et al. Systems training for emotional predictability and problem solving (STEPPS) for outpatients with borderline personality disorder: a randomized controlled trial and 1-year follow-up. *Am J Psychiatry.* 2008; 165: 468-478.

[24] Tyrer P, Sensky T, Mitchard S. Principles of nidotherapy in the treatment of persistent mental and personality disorders. *Psychother Psychosom.* 2003; 72: 350-356.

[25] Tyrer P, Bajaj P. Nidotherapy: making the environment do the therapeutic work. *Adv Psychiatr Treat.* 2005; 11: 232-238.

[26] Spencer SJ, Rutter D, Tyrer P. Integration of nidotherapy into the management of mental illness and antisocial personality: a qualitative study. *Int J Soc Psychiatry.* 2010; 56(1): 50-59.

[27] Ranger M, Tyrer P, Miloseska K, et al. Cost-effectiveness of nidotherapy for comorbid personality disorder and severe mental illness: randomized controlled trial. *Epidemiol Psichiatr Soc.* 2009; 18(2): 128-136.

In: Borderline Personality Disorder in Older Adults   ISBN: 978-1-63482-221-3
Editors: A. Hategan, J. A. Bourgeois, G. L. Xiong   © 2015 Nova Science Publishers, Inc.

Chapter 11

PHARMACOTHERAPY

Barbara J. Kocsis[1,], MD and Lorin M. Scher[2], MD*

[1]Psychiatry Resident,
Department of Psychiatry and Behavioral Sciences
University of California, at Davis, School of Medicine, CA, US
[2]Health Sciences Assistant Clinical Professor
Director, Emergency Psychiatry, Psychosomatic Medicine Service
Department of Psychiatry & Behavioral Sciences
University of California, at Davis, CA, US

Pharmacological interventions are common in geriatric borderline personality disorder (BPD) and require specific attention to age- and illness-specific considerations. The authors review the current literature on pharmacological treatment of BPD, emphasizing the considerations of age and psychiatric comorbidity. For practicality, pharmacological agents are grouped according to common mechanisms of action and symptom- and syndrome-specific classifications.

INTRODUCTION

Although the specific manifestations of BPD may shift over the lifespan, it remains a distressing affliction for many patients into their later years. It is generally held that the primary thrust of treatment for BPD is psychotherapy, and that pharmacology plays an adjunctive role. Indeed, the available literature thus far does not support the use of any single pharmacological agent for the treatment of BPD. No medications investigated have led to a reduction of overall BPD severity or improvement in general functioning [1], and none have a U.S. Food & Drug Administration (FDA) indication for treatment of BPD. Instead, medication therapies are typically aimed at specific symptom clusters within the disorder, or at other comorbid psychiatric conditions. Guidance for the treatment of older adults with BPD

* Corresponding author: bjkocsis@ucdavis.edu

is particularly scarce, as the vast majority of available literature examining both pharmacotherapy for BPD and the disorder in general were conducted using younger subjects.

GENERAL PRINCIPLES OF PHARMACOTHERAPY IN BORDERLINE PERSONALITY DISORDER

The goals of pharmacological intervention in BPD are to improve functioning and to enable participation in psychotherapy, to provide additional control over dangerous behaviors, and to treat comorbid mood and anxiety disorders. Common symptom targets in BPD are shown in Figure 11-1.

Impulsivity and self-harm behaviors

Affective instability and mood lability

Depressed mood

Psychosis and "micropsychotic" events

Dissociation

Anger and aggression

Comorbid mood and anxiety disorders

Figure 11-1. Common Pharmacological Targets in Borderline Personality Disorder.

An additional area of importance in prescribing for patients with BPD is setting reasonable expectations. Patients with BPD are prone to "black and white" or "all or nothing" thinking, and patient expectations can range widely from believing a drug may be useless and/or harmful, to considering it to be a panacea. Many patients will have tried several medications in the past, and thus may have a greater awareness of side effects, and/or may be hesitant to try a new agent. Interestingly, multiple medication trials for BPD have noted particularly robust placebo effects [2], which may be an indication of the significance of patient expectations among this population. Generally, it is useful for the clinician to emphasize that medication treatment will be one component of a larger treatment plan, in order to help these patients avoid pinning their hopes on medications alone. Frankly discussing potential side effects and offering anticipatory guidance about how these might be addressed may also be helpful.

Lastly, the clinician must keep in mind safety concerns when treating BPD patients with pharmacotherapy. This population frequently experiences suicidal ideation, and commonly engages in suicidal or parasuicidal behaviors. The clinician must always weigh the risks of toxicity in overdose when selecting medications. Patients with BPD are also at high risk for comorbid substance use disorders, and thus clinicians must exercise caution before prescribing addictive medications.

SPECIAL CONSIDERATIONS WHEN PRESCRIBING FOR OLDER ADULTS WITH BORDERLINE PERSONALITY DISORDER

In older adults, comorbid neurocognitive disorders can be common, and it may be prudent to first perform a formal cognitive assessment and decisional capacity assessment for specific clinical interventions before making further treatment decisions, as well as a baseline medical work-up.

The specifics of how BPD evolves over the lifetime, and how pharmacological agents may be best utilized, are important areas that necessitate further research. A small number of studies examining the natural course of BPD over the lifetime have found that certain symptoms seem to decline starting sometime between ages 30-40 [3-6]. As described earlier in Chapter 4, it appears that impulsivity-related, "active behaviors" (e.g., cutting, suicide attempts, comorbid substance abuse) decline, but affective-related features (e.g., chronic feelings of emptiness, dysphoria, evocation of strong countertransference) persist [3-6]. However, it has also been questioned if these effects are due to a possible failure of the diagnostic criteria to adequately describe BPD in older persons, or if psychiatrists may be hesitant to diagnose BPD in this age group [5]. Also see Chapter 2 for further details on personality and aging.

Pharmacological treatment for the older adult with BPD comes with further complicating factors (See Figure 11-2). The body undergoes changes with age that affect pharmacokinetics, including changes in serum protein levels, and in volume of distribution due to altered ratios of lean body weight to body fat. Reductions in hepatic and renal function occur naturally with aging, and many common medical problems such as diabetes mellitus or hypertension can lead to additional organ dysfunction. It is thus essential for the prescribing clinician to obtain an accurate medical history and baseline laboratory evaluation prior to starting new medication. The clinician should keep in mind that older adults may require substantially lower doses than their younger counterparts, and that a drug may be at an appropriate dose despite an apparently "subtherapeutic" drug level. The long-known adage "start low and go slow" regarding dosing is a wise strategy.

Impaired drug metabolism and altered pharmacokinetics

Comorbid systemic medical problems

Increased susceptibility to "deliriogenic" effects of medications

Increased fall risk

Polypharmacy

Compliance problems due to declining memory and mobility

Figure 11-2. Common Factors Affecting Use of Medications in Older Adults.

Older persons are at increased risk of adverse drug events, and common manifestations of these events include orthostatic hypotension, falls, and delirium. These risks are compounded by polypharmacy, which is common among older persons due to the increasing burden of medical illness with age. Polypharmacy increases the risk of drug-drug interactions and can result in prohibitively complex dosing schedules for the older adult. A clinician might consider setting specific treatment goals, or even a medication end-date, to ensure that unhelpful therapies are stopped. Several tools, such as the Beers criteria and STOPP (Screening Tool in Older Persons for Potentially Inappropriate Prescriptions) criteria are available to aid the clinician in identifying particularly high-risk medications [7]. Practical barriers to treatment adherence must also be addressed, including memory, mobility, and financial constraints. Strategies for prescribing for older individuals are listed in Figure 11-3.

Carefully weigh risks/benefits before starting any new drug

Obtain a thorough medical history

Obtain appropriate baseline laboratory tests (e.g. liver and kidney function)

Start low, go slow

Set therapeutic goal(s) and stop medication if not met

Avoid high-risk medications

Start one medication at a time, if possible

Arrange close follow-up whenever starting any new medication

Consider lowering the doses of or stopping other non-essential medications

Communicate frequently with a patient's primary care physician and other care providers

Figure 11-3. Safe Prescribing Strategies for Older Adults.

SPECIFIC PHARMACOLOGICAL THERAPIES FOR BORDERLINE PERSONALITY DISORDER IN OLDER ADULTS

Currently, there are no studies that specifically address the use of pharmacotherapies in older adults with BPD. However, the ensuing discussion is a summary of current evidence regarding the use of pharmacotherapy in persons with BPD, with particular emphasis on the older adults. It is difficult to draw firm conclusions from available data for several reasons, including few randomized controlled trials, small study sizes, limited variety of pharmacological agents studied, and study subjects drawn from predominantly young, outpatient populations.

Antidepressants

Antidepressant medications are commonly prescribed to patients with BPD in an attempt to target dysphoria and feelings of emptiness. However, small trials examining *fluoxetine, fluvoxamine, phenelzine*, and *mianserin* found no significant effects on these symptoms, and it appeared that fluoxetine may even worsen depression in this population [1]. One study of *fluvoxamine* (N=38) suggested possible improvement in affective instability, though the study may have been underpowered [1]. A single small (N=59) study of *amitriptyline* did find a modest effect in the reduction of depression [1], though this agent must be used with caution in older adults with BPD, given the deliriogenic anticholinergic effects and the significant toxicity of *tricyclic antidepressants* in overdose. Overall, antidepressants have thus far also failed to show any beneficial effect on anxiety, anger, impulsivity, dissociation, or overall BPD severity. A 2010 Cochrane review and several subsequent meta-analyses concluded that there is currently scant evidence to support the use of antidepressants in BPD, though they may be helpful for comorbid mood and anxiety disorders [1, 2, 8].

Mood Stabilizers

In contrast to antidepressant therapy, treatment with mood stabilizers seems to confer positive effects on several symptom clusters within BPD. In general, *valproate, lamotrigine, topiramate,* and *carbamazepine* have been the most studied. None of these mood stabilizers showed any significant impact on overall BPD severity, avoidance of abandonment, or psychotic symptoms, however.

Valproate/Divalproex sodium. A few small studies suggest that treatment with valproate leads to a reduction in interpersonal problems and anger in BPD. Additionally, it may also improve symptoms of depression. However, valproate had no effect on impulsivity, and one study showed a trend towards worsened suicidal ideation, though the effect was not statistically significant [1]. Though the data is too limited to draw a solid conclusion, valproate may be most helpful for the BPD patient who is particularly limited by irritability, but who is not strongly impulsive. In older adults, valproate should be started at low doses and titrated up slowly due to decreased elimination and increased experience of somnolence. Patients require baseline liver associated enzymes assessment with a repeat in 6 months, and baseline complete blood count with periodic reassessment to monitor for thrombocytopenia [9]. Serum ammonia may be monitored as valproate may be associated with hyperammonemia (which may present as delirium) in the absence of hepatocellular injury. The standard "therapeutic range" of 50-100 µg/mL for valproate is more validated for treatment of bipolar disorder and epilepsy; patients with BPD, especially if older, tend to require smaller doses of the medication. Despite the hypothesized neuroprotective properties of divalproex treatment, several studies have shown an association between valproate use and brain atrophy with cognitive impairment, but the long-term clinical effects of these changes still remain unknown [10].

Lamotrigine. Limited data imply that lamotrigine may improve impulsivity, affective instability, and anger in BPD, though it did not impact overall BPD severity [1]. It is feasible that this agent may be most helpful in BPD patients who are particularly impulsive or volatile. Patients should have baseline laboratory evaluation of renal and hepatic function prior to initiation of lamotrigine. Lamotrigine tends to be well-tolerated. Dosing for older individuals is generally the same as standard adult dosing, unless significant renal or hepatic impairment is present. The most concerning potential side effect is a rash, which can progress to Stevens-Johnson Syndrome; any appearance of rash should lead to prompt lamotrigine discontinuation and medical evaluation [9].

Topiramate. A few studies of topiramate showed a reduction in BPD-related impulsivity, anger, and anxiety [1]. A clinician may consider this agent for the anxious patient with BPD, especially since other anxiolytics (chiefly benzodiazepines) carry multiple risks (See discussion below). Additionally, topiramate was consistently associated with modest weight loss, and may be a good choice for the overweight patient. This agent should be initiated at 25 mg/day (half of adult dose) in older adults due to decreased renal clearance, with titration by 25 mg/day weekly. Patients should have baseline laboratory tests assessing renal function and electrolytes, with periodic reassessment (9). Patients should be counseled regarding the risk of renal stones; patients with a history of renal stones should not receive topiramate.

Others. The few studies that examined the use of *carbamazepine* in patients with BPD found no significant differences in any of the symptom clusters examined [1]. Currently, no studies are available assessing *lithium* for patients with BPD.

Antipsychotics

Antipsychotic agents are commonly employed in the treatment of BPD. Although there are no direct comparison studies, contemporary clinical practices for the care of older patients prefer the use of second-generation ("atypical") over first-generation ("typical") antipsychotics, mostly because of the increased concerns of adverse events such as parkinsonism and tardive dyskinesia with first-generation agents. While antipsychotics have been demonstrated to cause weight gain in all age groups, the magnitude of weight gain may be less concerning in older than in younger patients [11]. Although antipsychotics have been associated with an increased risk of developing diabetes mellitus, the risk may also be lower in older than younger patients [11]. Metabolic syndrome is another serious adverse event associated with antipsychotic use, particularly second-generation antipsychotics. Metabolic syndrome has not been particularly studied in geriatric patients, but it warrants special attention with recommended monitoring (e.g., weight/body mass index, blood pressure, fasting glucose/HbA1c, and fasting lipids) at baseline, three months, and annually thereafter [9, 11]. Use of an alternative medication is indicated if a patient develops metabolic syndrome. Generally, when prescribing antipsychotics for older adults with BPD, it is important to remember that many of these agents have side effects that may be particularly harmful to this population, including worsening of parkinsonism, orthostatic hypotension, and falls. Additionally, several drug regulatory agencies, including the U.S. FDA, have issued specific warnings for using antipsychotic medication in geriatric patients with dementia, as these agents have been shown to increase mortality in that population [9]. Generally, effective doses of both first- and second-generation antipsychotics are lower for BPD than psychotic disorders, and lower still in older BPD patients due to age-related pharmacokinetic and pharmacodynamic changes. The following antipsychotics have been the most studied in BPD.

First-Generation Antipsychotics

Butyrophenones. Haloperidol showed a benefit in reducing anger in BPD patients, but had no effect on impulsivity. Interestingly, it did not have a significant effect on psychotic symptoms [1]. As other agents discussed here have also been found to address anger with less risk of side effects, haloperidol may not be a first-line choice for the management of anger in BPD patients.

Thioxanthenes. Thiothixene did not show any beneficial effects on symptoms of BPD in limited studies. A single study demonstrated that *flupenthixol* decanoate-treated patients engaged in less suicidal behavior, though the study was conducted in younger patients [1].

Second-Generation Antipsychotics

Olanzapine. A few studies demonstrated that olanzapine improves anxiety, affective instability, anger, and psychotic symptoms among patients with BPD [1]. However, no effect was seen on avoidance of abandonment, identity disturbance, and impulsivity. Olanzapine is one of the few agents for which adverse effects have been reported in BPD patients. A small number of studies identified olanzapine as *worsening* suicidal ideation in patients with BPD, and the studies also showed trends suggesting that olanzapine treated patients had more suicidal and self-mutilating behavior [1]. Again, these findings may be biased by patient selection as some studies do not include patients who are actively suicidal. As it is highly sedating, a low starting dose of 2.5 mg daily is recommended in geriatric patients.

Aripiprazole. Available data suggest this agent reduces interpersonal problems, impulsivity, anger, and psychotic symptoms. Additionally, a non-significant trend indicated aripiprazole might reduce self-mutilating behavior. Aripiprazole may improve depression and anxiety in BPD patients as well [1]. Generally, aripiprazole is not sedating and requires no adjustment for reduced hepatic or renal function [9].

Quetiapine. One of the latest randomized, double-blind, placebo-controlled trials for BPD compared moderate- (300 mg daily) and low-dose (150 mg daily) quetiapine vs. placebo in 95 participants with BPD (mean age 30.1±8.8 years) over 8 weeks [12]. Among those who completed the study, 82% of the 150 mg/day group, 74% of the 300 mg/day group, and 48% in the placebo group responded to treatment. Response was defined as a reduction of 50% or more on the Zanarini Rating Scale for BPD symptoms total score [12]. There was higher drop-out rate in the mid-dose group due to side effects, especially sedation [12]. The agent did not appear to reduce impulsivity. A number of open-label, non-randomized studies also suggested that quetiapine may provide some benefit, though these results are more difficult to interpret given their design [8]. Quetiapine has notable anticholinergic effects and commonly causes orthostatic hypotension and sedation, and thus should be started at very low doses, such as 12.5 or 25 mg nightly.

Others. A number of studies showed that *ziprasidone* had no effect on BPD symptoms [1]. A few open-label, non-randomized studies and case series suggest possible benefit from *clozapine, risperidone, and paliperidone* [13-16].

Other Medication Classes

A few small studies have examined *omega-3 fatty acids* for treatment of BPD symptoms, and found statistically significant reductions in suicidal ideation and depression. No effect was seen for impulsivity, and patients possibly experienced worsened self-mutilation, though this effect was not statistically significant [1]. A single very small double-blind, placebo-controlled study of low- and mid-dose *naltrexone* (50 to 200 mg/day) found a trend toward reduction of dissociation in patients with BPD, although the study was too small for the effect to reach statistical significance [17]. Currently, evidence examining the use of *anxiolytics and hypnotics* in BPD is scant. It is a long-held belief that benzodiazepines are problematic due to potential for dependence and because they are thought to be disinhibiting in BPD [18, 19], although more research is needed. Generally, benzodiazepines are not recommended in geriatric patients with BPD because of risk of delirium and falls. There are no studies addressing the use of *buspirone* in BPD.

Evidence examining use of amphetamine-derived *psychostimulants* in BPD is also lacking, and is limited to two very small studies of comorbid attention deficit hyperactivity disorder and BPD in adolescents [20]. There is a small but growing movement examining the use of stimulants in older adults as a treatment for apathy in depression and other disorders [21], but not in BPD. Clinicians wishing to try a psychostimulant for an older patient with BPD must consider risks of disinhibition, addiction, worsening of psychotic/micropsychotic features, and any medical risks relevant to the patient (e.g., cardiac risks). There are no studies examining *modafinil,* the alpha-blocker *prazosin*, or cognition enhancers such as *donepezil* and *memantine* in patients with BPD.

In summary, Table 11-1 lists the evidence from higher quality studies addressing pharmacotherapy in BPD [1, 12]. However, these studies are based on adult population and not those aged 65 years or older. In the 2010 Cochrane review of pharmacotherapy for BPD, the reported mean participants' ages ranged from 21.7 to 38.6 years, with 14 of the 28 studies having a mean age below 30 years [1].

Table 11-1. Summary of Evidence Base for Efficacious Pharmacological Treatments in Borderline Personality Disorder [1, 12]

	Avoidance of Abandonment	Interpersonal Problems	Identity Disturbance	Impulsivity	Suicidality	Self-Injury	Affective Instability	Chronic Feelings of emptiness	Anger/ Aggression	Psychosis	Overall BPD Severity
Fluvoxamine				0			+		0		
Valproate		+		0	0/-				+		
Lamotrigine				+			+		+		0
Topiramate		+		+					+	0	
Quetiapine[12]		+	+	0			+/-		+		+
Olanzapine	0		0	0	-	0/-	+	0	+	+	0
Aripiprazole		+		+		0/+			+	+	
Omega-3 FA				0	+	0/-					

Note: (+): Beneficial effect; (-): Harmful effect; (0): No significant effect; (blank): Not yet studied. Most of the data was gathered from reference (1). Quetiapine information was based on reference (12). Studies are based on adult population and not older adults **aged ≥65 years.**

Case 1 – Mrs. M

Mrs. M, a 68-year-old obese woman, was admitted to a psychiatric hospital after an argument at home with her niece. During the argument, Mrs. M threw and broke several dishes. Frightened and angered by her aunt, Mrs. M's niece left the home. Mrs. M felt deeply ashamed of her behavior and distressed that her niece had left; her feelings of emptiness and self-reproach peaked, and she impulsively swallowed twenty 300 mg tablets of gabapentin, which were prescribed to her for diabetic neuropathy.

While in the hospital, the psychiatrist noted that Mrs. M struggled in maintaining connections with others and often "split" hospital staff into "good" and "bad" people. She displayed dramatic shifts in her affect when she felt slighted, and frequently expressed rage towards hospital staff and other patients that was particularly disruptive during therapy groups. The psychiatrist felt that Mrs. M would benefit from the hospital's therapy groups, and met with her to discuss how starting a medication might improve her ability to participate.

The psychiatrist selected topiramate, slowly titrated to 50 mg twice daily, to target Mrs. M's impulsivity and anger, with the additional hope that it may help her to lose weight and improve glycemic control. She tolerated topiramate well, and staff noted an improvement in her ability to participate in therapy, though she still struggled at times. Additionally, she lost 7 lbs. over 3 months and had a 1.5%-point improvement on her subsequent HbA1c.

Case 2 – Mr. B

Mr. B, a 78-year-old man with a long history of BPD, resided in a skilled nursing facility due to physical decline and difficulty recovering from a hip fracture suffered one year previously. Though Mr. B did not self-injure as much as he used to, he still struggled with strong negative affect and feelings of emptiness and anger when his family left at the end of a visit, or when he felt the physical therapist "pushed him too hard." As his distress had always been "situational," last year his primary care physician had prescribed a short-acting benzodiazepine for him to take as needed during distressing moments. Unfortunately, the medication had caused him to fall and thus led to his hip fracture. Recently, his family had been visiting less often, and his dysphoria and anxiety surrounding their departures escalated to the point that he began intermittently hearing voices and head-banging.

The consulting psychiatrist evaluated Mr. B, and after a thorough medical work-up concluded that these symptoms were attributable to his long-standing personality disorder. After a discussion of risks and benefits, Mr. B was started on 2 mg of aripiprazole, subsequently increased to 5 mg every morning with the goal of reducing impulsivity, psychotic symptoms, self-injury, and any underlying depression. The psychiatrist felt that aripiprazole, as it is less sedating, was a good choice given Mr. B's history of falls. Mr. B experienced a reduction in the frequency and severity of his episodes of acting out, and staff noted his participation in physical therapy also improved.

KEY POINTS: PHARMACOTHERAPY

- Although pharmacology plays an important adjunctive role, the primary treatment for BPD remains the psychotherapeutic interventions.
- No medications studied thus far have led to a reduction of overall BPD severity or improvement in general functioning, and none have an FDA indication for treatment of BPD.
- The goals of pharmacologic intervention in BPD are to improve functioning to enable participation in psychotherapy, to provide additional control over dangerous symptoms, and to treat comorbid mood and anxiety disorders.
- Older adults with BPD present similar pharmacotherapeutic treatment challenges as their younger counterparts, and in addition are subject to several physical changes with aging that put them at increased risk for adverse drug events.
- Generally, antidepressants are marginally helpful in BPD, and more robust effects have been found for treatment with mood stabilizers and low doses of second-generation antipsychotics.
- More research specifically examining the use of pharmacotherapy in older patients with BPD is greatly needed.

REFERENCES

[1]   Stoffers J, Vollm BA, Rucker G, Timmer A, Huband N, Lieb K. Pharmacological interventions for borderline personality disorder. *Cochrane Database Syst Rev.* 2010(6):Cd005653.

[2]   Vita A, De Peri L, Sacchetti E. Antipsychotics, antidepressants, anticonvulsants, and placebo on the symptom dimensions of borderline personality disorder: a meta-analysis of randomized controlled and open-label trials. *J Clin Psychopharmacol.* 2011; 31(5): 613-624.

[3]   Grant BF, Chou SP, Goldstein RB, et al. Prevalence, correlates, disability, and comorbidity of DSM-IV borderline personality disorder: results from the Wave 2 National Epidemiologic Survey on Alcohol and Related Conditions. *J Clin Psychiatry.* 2008; 69(4): 533-545.

[4]   De Moor MH, Distel MA, Trull TJ, Boomsma DI. Assessment of borderline personality features in population samples: is the Personality Assessment Inventory-Borderline Features scale measurement invariant across sex and age? *Psychol Assess.* 2009; 21(1): 125-130.

[5]   Ullrich S, Coid J. The age distribution of self-reported personality disorder traits in a household population. *J Pers Disord.* 2009; 23(2): 187-200.

[6]   Arens EA, Stopsack M, Spitzer C, et al. Borderline personality disorder in four different age groups: a cross-sectional study of community residents in Germany. *J Pers Disord.* 2013; 27(2): 196-207.

[7]   Pretorius RW, Gataric G, Swedlund SK, Miller JR. Reducing the risk of adverse drug events in older adults. *Am Fam Physician.* 2013; 87(5): 331-336.

[8] Ripoll LH. Psychopharmacologic treatment of borderline personality disorder. *Dialogues Clin Neurosci.* 2013; 15(2): 213-224.

[9] Lexicomp Online™. 2014; https://online.lexi.com. Accessed 10/09/2014.

[10] Fleisher AS, Truran D, Mai JT, et al. Chronic divalproex sodium use and brain atrophy in Alzheimer disease. *Neurology.* 2011; 77(13): 1263-1271.

[11] Chahine LM, Acar D, Chemali Z. The elderly safety imperative and antipsychotic usage. *Harv Rev Psychiatry.* 2010; 18(3): 158-172.

[12] Black DW, Zanarini MC, Romine A, et al. Comparison of Low and Moderate Dosages of Extended-Release Quetiapine in Borderline Personality Disorder: A Randomized, Double-Blind, Placebo-Controlled Trial. *Am J Psychiatry.* 2014 Jun 27. doi: 10.1176/appi.ajp.2014.13101348. [Epub ahead of print].

[13] Beri A, Boydell J. Clozapine in borderline personality disorder: a review of the evidence. *Ann Clin Psychiatry.* 2014; 26(2): 139-144.

[14] Carrasco JL, Palomares N, Marsa MD. Effectiveness and tolerability of long-acting intramuscular risperidone as adjuvant treatment in refractory borderline personality disorder. *Psychopharmacology (Berl).* 2012; 224(2): 347-348.

[15] Rocca P, Marchiaro L, Cocuzza E, Bogetto F. Treatment of borderline personality disorder with risperidone. *J Clin Psychiatry.* 2002; 63(3): 241-244.

[16] Bellino S, Bozzatello P, Rinaldi C, Bogetto F. Paliperidone ER in the treatment of borderline personality disorder: A pilot study of efficacy and tolerability. *Depress Res Treat.* 2011; 2011: 680194. doi: 10.1155/2011/680194. Epub 2011 Aug 4.

[17] Schmahl C, Kleindienst N, Limberger M, et al. Evaluation of naltrexone for dissociative symptoms in borderline personality disorder. *Int Clin Psychopharmacol.* 2012; 27(1): 61-68.

[18] Cowdry RW, Gardner DL. Pharmacotherapy of borderline personality disorder. Alprazolam, carbamazepine, trifluoperazine, and tranylcypromine. *Arch Gen Psychiatry.* 1988; 45(2): 111-119.

[19] Gardner DL, Cowdry RW. Alprazolam-induced dyscontrol in borderline personality disorder. *Am J Psychiatry.* 1985; 142(1): 98-100.

[20] Asherson P, Young AH, Eich-Hochli D, Moran P, Porsdal V, Deberdt W. Differential diagnosis, comorbidity, and treatment of attention-deficit/hyperactivity disorder in relation to bipolar disorder or borderline personality disorder in adults. *Curr Med Res Opin.* 2014; 30(8): 1657-1672.

[21] Sinita E, Coghill D. The use of stimulant medications for non-core aspects of ADHD and in other disorders. *Neuropharmacology.* 2014; 87C: 161-172.

In: Borderline Personality Disorder in Older Adults   ISBN: 978-1-63482-221-3
Editors: A. Hategan, J. A. Bourgeois, G. L. Xiong   © 2015 Nova Science Publishers, Inc.

Chapter 12

SOMATIC AND NOVEL PHARMACOLOGICAL TREATMENTS

Gary M. Hasey[1,], MD, MSc*
and Glen L. Xiong[2], MD, CMD

[1]Associate Professor, Psychiatry
Faculty of Health Sciences, Department of Psychiatry
and Behavioural Neurosciences, School of Biomedical Engineering,
Department of Electrical and Computer Engineering, McMaster University
Director of the Donald and Lillian Mair rTMS Laboratory
and the ECT program, St Joseph's Hospital, Hamilton, ON, Canada
[2]Health Sciences Associate Clinical Professor, Psychiatry
Department of Psychiatry and Behavioral Sciences,
University of California, at Davis, CA, US

Borderline personality disorder (BPD) is often comorbid with major depressive disorder and associated with more frequent hospitalizations, more extensive use of psychiatric resources and greater treatment-resistance compared to other personality disorders.

Discussion of the entire range of somatic and pharmacological options that might be considered in the treatment-resistant patient with BPD is beyond the scope of this short chapter. We therefore limit our review to those more novel treatment modalities that we believe are either the most viable or the most topical for BPD given the information available at this time. We will focus on the treatment of the complex, seriously ill geriatric patient, typically diagnosed with comorbid psychiatric pathology and requiring treatment in an institutional setting.

In the section on somatic therapies we discuss electroconvulsive therapy (ECT), repetitive transcranial magnetic stimulation (rTMS) and deep brain stimulation (DBS). In the section on pharmacotherapies we discuss ketamine infusion and L-methylfolate. We conclude that ECT, rTMS and L-methylfolate could be useful treatment modalities for the complicated patient with BPD, particularly if there is comorbid major depressive

---
* Corresponding author: Mood Disorders Program, St Joseph's Healthcare, 100 West 5th Street, Hamilton, Ontario, L8N 3K7, Canada, ghasey@sympatico.ca

disorder. DBS is highly invasive and the evidence supporting its utility for major depressive disorder is being questioned. The beneficial effect of ketamine is brief; the drug must be administered intravenously and can produce dissociation and cardiovascular effects that may be problematic for the geriatric patient with BPD.

INTRODUCTION

There is a paucity of high quality somatic and novel pharmacological treatment studies of patients with BPD in the geriatric age group. Although there is some question about whether the syndromatic presentation of BPD in the older patient is identical to that of younger adults [1], as the illness is life-long, it is likely that the treatment histories will be similar. Compared with other types of personality pathology, BPD is associated with an earlier age of first treatment, a higher number of hospitalizations and greater likelihood of treatment with complex pharmacological combinations [2]. In addition, BPD is commonly comorbid with depressive illness [3]. For this reason many of the pharmacological and somatic treatments proposed for BPD are those employed in the management of the affective disorders. Both BPD and late-life depression are often difficult to treat [2, 4], and the disappointing results lead to relatively frequent consideration of ECT and highlight the need for new treatment options. In this chapter we briefly review the utility of ECT as well as some of the newer somatic and pharmacological therapies that might be considered in the treatment-resistant geriatric patient with BPD.

SOMATIC THERAPIES

Electroconvulsive Therapy (ECT)

Although the role of ECT in the treatment of BPD in the absence of other comorbidity is not clear [5], there is little question about the value of ECT in the treatment of major depressive disorder, particularly among the geriatric patients where remission rates of 90% (compared with 70% for those aged 45 or younger) are reported [6].

It has been suggested that the symptoms of BPD may improve or remit when comorbid major depressive disorder is treated [3]. However, in a study of 16 younger patients treated with ECT, borderline personality symptoms did not change significantly even though depressive symptoms were improved [7].

In contrast, the symptoms of major depressive disorder improve substantially after ECT in patients with BPD, though to a lesser extent than seen in depressed patients without comorbid BPD. In a prospective study of 139 depressed patients treated with ECT, those with no personality pathology, or with personality disorders other than BPD, showed decreases in depression rating scale scores of 70% and 68%, respectively, and remission rates of 70% and 56%, respectively, compared with only 47% decrease in depression scores and remission rate of 22% in those with BPD [8]. In this study the BPD subjects were significantly younger (mean age 32.7 years) than the other two groups (mean age 54.4 years). Although, for all subjects taken together, age was negatively correlated with the post-ECT Hamilton

Depression Rating Scale scores, the poorer outcome in the BPD group was not accounted for by this age difference.

Several other studies support the finding that BPD is associated with generally poorer outcome in patients treated with ECT. The authors of a review of 13 studies addressing the effect of personality pathology on the ECT response concluded that, "the available data suggests that depression in these patients can be effectively treated with ECT. The depressed, borderline patient appears to have two distinct disorders, one which is responsive to ECT and the other which is not" [9].

Repetitive Transcranial Magnetic Stimulation (rTMS)

Although there are no studies of rTMS in geriatric patients with BPD, the effect of rTMS on BPD has been examined in younger subjects. A 22-year-old female with BPD reported improved mood and decreased impulsivity after treatment with rTMS [10] and 4 women with depression, fibromyalgia, and BPD experienced greatly reduced physical pain after true but not sham rTMS [11]. There is only a single sham controlled trial where subjects with BPD (and no other comorbidity) received true (N=5) or sham (N=4) rTMS. The investigators observed significantly greater reduction in anger and affective instability after true compared with sham treatment [12]. rTMS has been much more extensively studied as an antidepressant treatment. A very large (N=190) sham-controlled prospective study confirmed the efficacy of rTMS in younger depressed subjects [13].

In the geriatric population, open label, uncontrolled trials report clinically significant response in 31-58% of those treated [14, 15] with better response being reported in the study using a longer series of rTMS treatments. Although two small prospective sham-controlled trials in depressed older subjects (N=24 and 20) failed to show a difference between true and sham rTMS treatments [16, 17], these studies were hampered by what was probably an insufficient number of treatments and very low magnetic pulse energy.

A much larger sham-controlled trial in geriatric patients (N=92) with evidence of "vascular depression" using a longer series of rTMS treatments and higher magnetic energy had better results. The investigators observed response and remission rates of 39.4% and 27.3% in the true rTMS group versus 6.9% and 3.5% in the sham group [18]. In these subjects the response was inversely correlated with age but directly correlated with frontal grey matter volume. The latter finding is in accordance with evidence that the magnetic field strength at the cortex surface is reduced if there is age-related brain shrinkage [19]. This is because the magnetic field strength decreases exponentially as the distance from the magnetic coil increases.

In the absence of data on rTMS in the geriatric population with BPD, we describe, below, a case of a middle aged adult patient to generate interest in studying outcomes in geriatric patients with similar clinical presentations. We expect that the response to this safe and non-invasive treatment would not differ substantially in the geriatric population; this would be an area for future clinical research.

Case 1 – Ms. A

Ms. A, a 41-year-old divorced woman with a long history of depression and BPD, was referred for rTMS after failed trials of at least 7 antidepressant medications. She had been hospitalized 3 times during the previous year because of suicidal ideation. She was adopted at an early age into an abusive family where she was frequently beaten and publically humiliated (e.g., after being caught masturbating). She considered herself bisexual. She cut her arms to alleviate stress as a teenager. As an adult she has been impulsive and, when under stress, sometimes saw magazine photo figures moving their lips. She first became seriously depressed after the birth of her first child. When she presented for assessment at the rTMS clinic she described depressed mood, poor self-esteem, interrupted sleep, low energy, impaired concentration, anhedonia, carbohydrate craving, a pessimistic outlook and frequent suicidal ideation. She received a course of 20 left sided 10 Hz rTMS. Her Hamilton Depression Rating Scale scores dropped from 28 to 16, which did not meet the typical threshold for clinically significant response (at least 50% improvement). Her Beck Depression Inventory score only dropped from 35 (severely depressed) to 21 (moderately depressed). Nonetheless, she reported substantial improvement in her ability to function at home. After 2 months she relapsed and returned for maintenance rTMS, which continued indefinitely. Most significantly, despite her past history of repeated hospitalizations, she has not required readmission during the last 3 years of follow-up at our clinic. Ms. A continues to receive maintenance rTMS, on average, every 2 weeks. Her Beck Depression Inventory scores remain in the moderately depressed range (low 20s) but she maintains that she feels much better since rTMS was started. Over the 3 year period of stability she gradually stopped taking mirtazapine because of weight gain but continued to take paroxetine 40 mg daily together with rTMS. Ms. A was on no other psychotropic medications and she does not receive any psychotherapy other than the supportive psychotherapy that is part of the rTMS program.

Deep Brain Stimulation (DBS)

DBS is still highly investigational. Although there is some evidence that DBS may be an effective treatment for medication-resistant major depression and other neuropsychiatric conditions [20], two studies of DBS for the treatment of major depressive disorder were halted by the U.S. Food & Drug Administration (FDA) after "failed futility analysis" [20]. Although the precise meaning of this term is not stated in the cited article, typically it can mean interim analysis suggests that the effect of the true intervention is not likely to exceed that of the sham intervention.

So far there are no studies of deep brain stimulation as a treatment for BPD in geriatric patients. A study of DBS of the fornix/hippocampus of 6 geriatric subjects with mild Alzheimer's disease resulted in "early and striking reversal of the impaired glucose utilization in the temporal and parietal lobes" [21]. However, only "possible improvements" of cognitive functioning were described. There is also a case report of a 49-year-old woman with comorbid major depressive disorder, bulimia nervosa, and BPD, who improved dramatically after bilateral implantation of stimulation electrodes in the inferior thalamic peduncle [22].

Table 12-1. Somatic Therapy for BPD and Major Depressive Disorder

Author	Sample size/Diagnosis/Age	Treatment/Design	Results
O'Connor et al. 2001 [6]	N=253 MDD Age: see results column	ECT open label	Remission by age: >65 =90% 46-64=89.8% <46=70%
Blais et al. 1998 [7]	N=16 MDD Mean age=55	ECT open label	Small decrease in BPD symptoms after ECT P=.06 BPD symptoms associated with poorer response
Feske et al. 2004 [8]	N=139 MDD +/- PD Mean age=58.3, 50.4, 37.7, respectively (see results column)	ECT open label	Remission rate by PDs: No PD=70% Non-BPD PD=56% BPD=22%
DeBattista & Mueller 2001 [9]	Review of 13 studies MDD+ BPD Ages not specified	ECT open label	MDD responds, BPD does not respond
Arbabi et al. 2013 [10]	N=1 BPD Age=22	rTMS X 10 open label	Improved mood and decreased impulsivity
Sampson et al. 2006 [11]	N=4 with MDD+BPD+FMA Age=39-51	rTMS partially sham controlled	Reduced pain after true but not sham
Cailhol et al. 2014 [12]	N=9 with BPD Age=22-45	rTMS X 10 randomized sham controlled	Decreased anger and affective instability True>sham
George et al. 2010 [13]	N=190 MDD Age=22-69	rTMS X 21+ randomized sham	Remission rate True=14.1% Sham=5.1%
Abraham et al. 2007 [14]	N=19 MDD Age>60	rTMS X 10 open label	6 responded, with mean of 31.6% decrease in depression scores
Hizli et al. 2013 [15]	N=65 MDD Age>60	rTMS X 18 open label	58% responded, 50% remitted
Manes et al. 2001 [16]	N=24 MDD Mean age=60.7	rTMS X 5 randomized sham controlled	True=Sham
Mosimann et al. 2004 [17]	N=20 MDD Mean age=62	rTMS X 10 randomized sham controlled	True=Sham
Jorge et al. 2008 [18]	N=92 "Vascular depression" Age>50 , mean=62-66	rTMS X 10 randomized sham controlled	Response/remission: True=39.4%/27.3% Sham=6.9%/3.5%
Laxton et al. 2010 [21]	N=6 Mild Alzheimer's disease Age=40-80	DBS Fornix/hippocampus open label	Reversed impaired glucose utilization on PET scanning, maintained at least 12 months, modest cognitive improvement
Jimenez et al. 2005 [22]	N=1 MDD + BPD + Bulimia Age=49	DBS inferior thalamic peduncle	Transient improvement of depression and global assessment of function scores with implantation but current off. Subsequent more sustained improvement with current on.

Note: BPD, Borderline personality disorder; DBS, Deep brain stimulation; ECT, Electroconvulsive therapy; FMA, Fibromyalgia; MDD, Major depressive disorder; PD, Personality disorder; rTMS, Repetitive transcranial magnetic stimulation.

Interestingly, there was significant improvement after implantation but before the electrodes were activated, suggesting either a very strong placebo effect or the potential beneficial effect of micro-damage (e.g., edema or inflammation) due to the surgical placement of electrodes in this region.

A placebo effect seems less likely in view of the observation that, after several months of sustained improvement, the patient relapsed during a blinded trial where the device was turned off without the subject's knowledge. These somatic treatment studies discussed in this section have been summarized in Table 12-1 [6-18, 21, 22].

ADVANCES IN PHARMACOLOGY

For the purposes of this chapter, we selectively discuss emerging medications currently used off-label in general psychiatry and not covered in the Chapter 11: Pharmacotherapy. As such, this chapter covers medications that may be applied for treatment of psychiatric comorbidities in BPD, particularly treatment-resistant depression. When BPD and depression are highly comorbid, BPD most often is the contributing factor to "treatment resistance." Nevertheless, treatment of the mood disorder (especially when severe) is often necessary before the patient can engage in outpatient combined non-pharmacological and medication treatment. As a complete review of the large number of investigational and alternative medications considered for treatment resistance (e.g., scopolamine, psychostimulants, memantine, riluzole, omega-3 fatty acids) is beyond the scope of this chapter, we focus on two novel medications that have gained considerable recent clinical attention and are likely to have the most clinical relevance to BPD: ketamine and L-methylfolate.

Ketamine

Based on case reports and small controlled studies, intravenous infusion of ketamine has gained increasing interest for off-label clinical use for treatment-resistant depression. Of note, ketamine infusion requires a period of inpatient monitoring and therefore is most often used for inpatients. Ketamine, thought to work as an antagonist at the N-methyl-D-aspartate (NMDA) receptor, may alleviate depressive symptoms in a matter of hours. Response to ketamine may be mediated by genetic factors. Carriers of the Val66Met single nucleotide polymorphism, which is associated with reduced brain-derived neurotrophic factor activity, seem to be poor responders [23]. A systematic review and meta-analysis of ketamine for the treatment of unipolar and bipolar depression found that this drug can induce significant acute and rapid reduction of depressive symptoms including suicidal ideation [23]. However, as most of the non-ECT studies examined ketamine effects after only a single infusion, it is unclear if the improvement can be maintained. According to this meta-analysis, the duration of the antidepressant effects may be as short as 2-3 days [23]. Also, most of the controlled studies have not specifically examined use of ketamine in patients older than age 65, although some studies did not exclude older adults. The authors of the review concluded that studies with repeat dosing to assess maintenance effects are warranted. The most rigorous study using ketamine involved a two-site randomized midazolam-controlled study that measured reduction of depressive symptoms using the Montgomery-Asberg Depression Rating Scale [24]. At 24 hours after treatment, response (defined as reduction of baseline Montgomery-Asberg Depression Rating Scale score by 50% or more) was 68% with ketamine compared to 28% for midazolam control. While generating much excitement, the study raises several questions about ketamine dose, patient selection and safety concerns including transient hypertension in patients with pre-existing cardiovascular disease, which could be problematic particularly in geriatric patients with BPD. Of concern for patients with BPD who may already have comorbid dissociation, dissociative symptoms have been reported in 18% (8 of 47 patients) of those treated with ketamine [25].

L-Methylfolate

Folate deficiency is associated with depression and with poor response to antidepressants. The biologically active form of folate that crosses the blood brain barrier is L-methylfolate. L-methylfolate is a co-factor for tetrahydrobiopterin, which is needed to activate tryptophan hydroxylase and tyrosine hydroxylase, the enzymes that synthesize the monoamines serotonin, dopamine, and norepinephrine. A multi-center L-methylfolate augmentation study conducted in partially or completely SSRI-resistant patients employed a two-trial placebo controlled, sequential, randomized design involving 148 outpatients (ages 18-65) who were on stable antidepressant treatment [26]. The first trial using 7.5 mg/day of L-methylfolate for 30 days followed by 15 mg/day for 30 days vs. placebo found that only the 15 mg/day was more effective than placebo, however the difference did not reach statistical difference (P=0.1). The second trial (N=75) comparing 15 mg/day for 60 days with placebo (for 30 days) demonstrated response rate of 32.3% in the active drug group compared to 14.6% for placebo. Response was defined as a reduction in Hamilton Depression Rating Scale scores of 50% or more. L-methylfolate was well tolerated with minimal side effects.

Table 12-2. Advances in Pharmacotherapy for Treatment-Resistant Depression

Drug/Author	Sample size/ Diagnosis/Age	Comments
Ketamine (meta-analysis) Fond et al. 2014 (23)	N=192 MDD N=34 BD Age=18-65	For overall depressive score, SMD =0.99 (95% CI -1.23 to -0.75, *P*<0.01); duration of ketamine effect was only assessed in 2 of 9 non-ECT studies and seemed to last 2-3 days; 3 of 4 studies found reduced suicidal thoughts
Ketamine (single intravenous infusion) Murrough et al. 2013 (24)	N=72 (2:1 ketamine vs. midazolam) Mean age= 46.9±12.8 (women) and 42.9±11.6 (men)	Two site-study, number needed to treat (NNT) was 2.8 for ketamine specific response; about half relapse within one week, 8 of 47 patients had dissociated symptoms, 2 subjects had to stop infusion due to blood pressure issues
L-methylfolate (for treatment resistant depression) Papakostas et al. 2012 (26)	N=148 (Trial 1) N=75 (Trial 2) Mean age=47.9±11.6 (Trial 1) Mean age=48.4±12.1	Trial 1 comparing placebo, 7.5 and 15 mg/day was negative. Trial 2 compared 15 mg/day for 30 days; antidepressants used were exclusively SSRIs; it is possible that longer treatment would lead to more responders as seen in STAR*D.

Note: BD, Bipolar depression; MDD, Major depressive disorder; SSRIs, Selective serotonin reuptake inhibitors; STAR*D, Sequenced treatment alternatives to relieve depression; SMD, Standardized mean difference.

Overall, it appears that patients with BPD would likely tolerate L-methylfolate quite well with minimum side effects. However, L-methylfolate is marketed as a "medical food" and, therefore, not regulated by the FDA. As such, it is not considered a pharmaceutical and is not covered by medical insurance companies. At the time of this writing, L-methylfolate costs up to USD150 for a 30-day supply. The pharmacotherapies discussed in this section are summarized in Table 12-2 [23, 24, 26].

Case 2 – Mr. B

Mr. B, a 68-year-old retired business executive, was admitted to hospital following a suicide attempt via wrist laceration. He had received multiple antidepressant treatment trials for depression and completed 15 sessions of ECT treatment prior to admission for severe depression and suicidal ideation. Mr. B was cooperative on interview. He disclosed that he was living with his daughter following his divorce 12 months ago. His ex-wife at that time was living with another man and would not speak to him, despite the fact that he had tried to contact her multiple times. He did not recall the events of his suicide attempt, except that he felt lonely because his daughter and the rest of her family went out for dinner with the patient's ex-wife.

A comorbid diagnosis of BPD was considered. Mr. B requested further ECT for his depression, despite the fact that he was not sure if he responded well to the first course of ECT.

After considering Mr. B's complex presentation, the team decided to defer ECT treatment for the time being. To the team's surprise, Mr. B did not strongly object to the team's refusal to provide ECT treatment. Instead, the treatment team offered the possible diagnosis of BPD to the patient based on his life history and current symptoms, citing that the patient had depression and comorbid BPD, and that, in addition to pharmacotherapy, non-pharmacological treatment should be explored.

The treatment team worked with Mr. B to identify his fantasy that he would reunite with his wife. He agreed to move in with roommate rather than return to live with his daughter. Several months later, he decided to return to the workforce. He continued outpatient psychiatric treatment and had not made a suicide attempt for at least 12 months after discharge. He is currently taking sertraline 100 mg/day and L-methylfolate 15 mg/day for treatment-resistant depression.

BPD may be a leading cause of treatment-resistant depression. Complicated pharmacotherapy is common in patients with BPD and they are often referred for ECT because of treatment resistance. In Mr. B's case, the diagnosis of BPD was strongly suspected. It is not uncommon that patients with BPD will "demand" ECT treatment. As discussed previously, BPD is associated with a poorer antidepressant response to ECT compared with those who receive either another personality disorder diagnosis or have no personality pathology [8].

KEY POINTS: SOMATIC AND NOVEL PHARMACOLOGICAL TREATMENTS

- ECT is an effective treatment for major depressive disorder but does little to improve the symptoms of BPD.
- Patients with comorbid major depressive disorder and BPD respond less well to ECT than those with no personality pathology or with personality disorders other than BPD.
- rTMS is clearly effective for major depressive disorder; patients with BPD may experience improved mood and decreased anger, affective instability and pain, but the evidence supporting this is still weak.
- DBS is highly investigational and the FDA has halted trials of DBS for major depressive disorder; a case study suggests DBS has beneficial effects in patients with comorbid major depressive disorder and BPD.
- Intravenous ketamine may have acute antidepressant effects in treatment-resistant patients but the beneficial effect may not last longer than 2-3 days.
- Ketamine may produce dissociative effects and acute hypertension that could be problematic in geriatric patients with BPD.
- L-methylfolate is well tolerated and, in doses of 15mg/day, may be a useful adjunctive treatment in those on antidepressant medications.
- Ketamine and L-methyfolate studies have not been specifically examined in patients aged 65 years or older.

REFERENCES

[1]   Rosowsky E, Gurian B. Borderline personality disorder in late life. *Int Psychogeriatr.* 1991; 3(1): 39-52.
[2]   Zanarini MC, Frankenburg FR, Khera GS, Bleichmar J. Treatment histories of borderline inpatients. *Compr Psychiatry.* 2001; 42(2): 144-150.
[3]   Gunderson JG, Elliott GR. The interface between borderline personality disorder and affective disorder. *Am J Psychiatry.* 1985; 142(3): 277-288.
[4]   Flint AJ. Treatment-resistant depression in late life. *CNS Spectr.* 2002; 7(10): 733-738.
[5]   Gagliardi JP, Krishnan RR. Evidence for the treatment of borderline personality disorder. *Psychopharmacol Bull.* 2003; 37(1): 30-46.
[6]   O'Connor MK, Knapp R, Husain M, et al. The influence of age on the response of major depression to electroconvulsive therapy: a C.O.R.E. Report. *Am J Geriatr Psychiatry.* 2001; 9(4): 382-390.
[7]   Blais MA, Matthews J, Schouten R, O'Keefe SM, Summergrad P. Stability and predictive value of self-report personality traits pre- and post-electroconvulsive therapy: a preliminary study. *Compr Psychiatry.* 1998; 39(4): 231-235.
[8]   Feske U, Mulsant BH, Pilkonis PA, et al. Clinical outcome of ECT in patients with major depression and comorbid borderline personality disorder. *Am J Psychiatry.* 2004; 161(11): 2073-2080.

[9]   DeBattista C, Mueller K. Is electroconvulsive therapy effective for the depressed patient with comorbid borderline personality disorder? *J ECT*. 2001; 17(2): 91-98.

[10] Arbabi M, Hafizi S, Ansari S, Oghabian MA, Hasani N. High frequency TMS for the management of Borderline Personality Disorder: a case report. *Asian J Psychiatr*. 2013; 6(6): 614-617.

[11] Sampson SM, Rome JD, Rummans TA. Slow-frequency rTMS reduces fibromyalgia pain. *Pain Med*. 2006; 7(2): 115-118.

[12] Cailhol L, Roussignol B, Klein R, et al. Borderline personality disorder and rTMS: a pilot trial. *Psychiatry Res*. 2014; 216(1): 155-157.

[13] George MS, Lisanby SH, Avery D, et al. Daily left prefrontal transcranial magnetic stimulation therapy for major depressive disorder: a sham-controlled randomized trial. *Arch Gen Psychiatry*. 2010; 67(5): 507-516.

[14] Abraham G, Milev R, Lazowski L, Jokic R, du Toit R, Lowe A. Repetitive transcranial magnetic stimulation for treatment of elderly patients with depression - an open label trial. *Neuropsychiatr Dis Treat*. 2007; 3(6): 919-924.

[15] Hizli Sayar G, Ozten E, Tan O, Tarhan N. Transcranial magnetic stimulation for treating depression in elderly patients. *Neuropsychiatr Dis Treat*. 2013; 9: 501-504.

[16] Manes F, Jorge R, Morcuende M, Yamada T, Paradiso S, Robinson RG. A controlled study of repetitive transcranial magnetic stimulation as a treatment of depression in the elderly. *Int Psychogeriatr*. 2001; 13(2): 225-231.

[17] Mosimann UP, Schmitt W, Greenberg BD, et al. Repetitive transcranial magnetic stimulation: a putative add-on treatment for major depression in elderly patients. *Psychiatry Res*. 2004; 126(2): 123-133.

[18] Jorge RE, Moser DJ, Acion L, Robinson RG. Treatment of vascular depression using repetitive transcranial magnetic stimulation. *Arch Gen Psychiatry*. 2008; 65(3): 268-276.

[19] Nahas Z, Li X, Kozel FA, et al. Safety and benefits of distance-adjusted prefrontal transcranial magnetic stimulation in depressed patients 55-75 years of age: a pilot study. *Depress Anxiety*. 2004; 19(4): 249-256.

[20] Cavuoto J. St. Jude Medical Struggles to Regain Traction in Neuromodulation Market. Neurotech Business Report. Available from: http://www.neurotechreports.com/pages/St_Jude_Medical_profile.html. Accessed November 5, 2014.

[21] Laxton AW, Tang-Wai DF, McAndrews MP, et al. A phase I trial of deep brain stimulation of memory circuits in Alzheimer's disease. *Ann Neurol* 2010; 68(4): 521-534.

[22] Jiménez F, Velasco F, Salin-Pascual R, et al. A patient with a resistant major depression disorder treated with deep brain stimulation in the inferior thalamic peduncle. *Neurosurgery*. 2005; 57(3): 585-593; discussion 585-593.

[23] Fond G, Loundou A, Rabu C, et al. Ketamine administration in depressive disorders: a systematic review and meta-analysis. *Psychopharmacology (Berl)*. 2014; 231(18): 3663-3676.

[24] Murrough JW, Iosifescu DV, Chang LC, et al. Antidepressant efficacy of ketamine in treatment-resistant major depression: a two-site randomized controlled trial. *Am J Psychiatry*. 2013; 170(10): 1134-1142.

[25] Rush AJ. Ketamine for treatment-resistant depression: ready or not for clinical use? *Am J Psychiatry.* 2013; 170(10): 1079-1081.

[26] Papakostas GI, Shelton RC, Zajecka JM, et al. L-methylfolate as adjunctive therapy for SSRI-resistant major depression: results of two randomized, double-blind, parallel-sequential trials. *Am J Psychiatry.* 2012; 169(12): 1267-1274.

In: Borderline Personality Disorder in Older Adults   ISBN: 978-1-63482-221-3
Editors: A. Hategan, J. A. Bourgeois, G. L. Xiong   © 2015 Nova Science Publishers, Inc.

Chapter 13

PALLIATIVE AND END-OF-LIFE CARE

Margaret W. Leung[1],, MD, MPH, Sheila Lahijani[2], MD
and Tua-Elisabeth Mulligan[3], MD*
[1]Palliative Medicine Fellow, Harvard Medical School,
Palliative Medicine, Boston, MA, US
[2]Psychosomatics Fellow,
Northwestern University Feinberg School of Medicine
Department of Psychiatry and Behavioral Sciences, Chicago, IL, US
[3]Psychiatry Resident, Department of Psychiatry
University of California San Francisco, San Francisco, CA, US

Palliative care is specialized care for patients with life-threatening medical illness that improves quality of life through addressing physical, psychosocial, emotional, and spiritual suffering. Palliative care transcends the patient-physician relationship to extend support for the family. It is appropriate at any age or stage of illness including patients who are receiving curative treatment. This chapter explores the medical and psychological discourse on end-of-life care, which incorporates symptom control and pain management, and also meaning-centered care with particular focus on older patients with psychiatric disorders including personality pathology. While this chapter offers a general overview and framework for understanding the complexities of managing these patients with empathic failures and existential issues, it does not represent a comprehensive review of the end-of-life care literature.

INTRODUCTION

The scope of palliative care practice includes managing symptoms such as pain or nausea, assisting with stress and coping related to serious disease, and counseling patients and families on advanced care planning [1]. In North America, hospice care refers to palliative care that treats patients with a prognosis of six months or less. Evidence suggests that

---

* Corresponding author: mwleung@mgh.harvard.edu

palliative care is cost effective, and improves patients' quality of life across multiple domains and satisfaction with care [2, 3].

Psychiatry overlaps considerably with palliative care through integrating physical, psychological, and social aspects of care. Psychiatrists are uniquely positioned to care for patients as they face serious medical illness that may exacerbate or complicate aspects of their mental health. Psychiatric disorders such as depression, anxiety, and delirium are common at the end of life [4]. In periods of crisis, patients' defenses that are adaptive and/or maladaptive peak. Geriatric patients with borderline personality disorder (BPD) and serious illness or at the end of life are likely to be at risk for psychiatric decompensation. Psychiatrists and other mental health professionals provide an important perspective on the psychological suffering that may arise for any patient struggling with fears, conflict, or guilt. They provide an important opportunity to build a therapeutic relationship and offer reparations for damages from patients' previous empathic failures [5].

FEATURES OF BORDERLINE PERSONALITY DISORDER IN PALLIATIVE CARE

Psychological suffering is nearly universal for patients experiencing life-limiting illness. Areas of potential suffering include pain and symptom control, making preparations for the end of life such as putting financial affairs in order, and achieving a sense of completion about one's life [6]. A patient's experience with terminal illness is shaped by a lifetime of characteristic defenses and coping mechanisms [7]. A unifying theme to consider for ill patients is the fear of abandonment which is particularly heightened at the end of life [8]. This fear resonates particularly with geriatric patients with BPD who have had a lifetime of fragile and fragmented relationships. Patients with BPD often do not have a secure attachment figure, and have difficulty integrating both "good" and "bad" qualities of others. They may attempt to secure attachments by displaying urgent and frequent care-seeking behaviors. Relationships with clinical staff are marked by constant confrontation and splitting as reactions to what they perceive as abandonment.

Friends and family can grow distant in the presence of the sick and dying. In situations where estranged family and/or friends may not want to be involved in the patient's care, there is a potential loss of not knowing what the patient's values and preferences for medical care decisions are. Consequently, identifying an individual who can advocate for the patient in situations where the patient is incapacitated to make decisions can be a challenge. The health care team may become the *de facto* "family" (although medical professionals cannot serve as surrogate consent agents) and may need to seek legal assistance in identifying a guardian on behalf of the patient. For older patients with BPD who do have some preserved relationships, serious illness changes these relationships. It can lead to a desire for deeper connection with loved ones. It also leads to worries about surviving family members such as the patient not wanting to be a burden as physical dependency increases. Palliative care team helps patients identify important people in their lives who can support them and encourage conversations to enhance relationships including saying goodbye. It also supports the family with anticipatory bereavement and in the period after death.

PALLIATIVE CARE APPROACHES TO GERIATRIC PATIENTS WITH BORDERLINE PERSONALITY DISORDER

The palliative care skillset for clinicians emphasizes patient-centered communication. This skill is useful for working with patients with BPD, with whom clear, consistent communication is particularly important. The "ask-tell-ask" format explores patient understanding of his or her medical situation, educates the patient, corrects misunderstandings, and has the patient explain back what was said and provides opportunities to ask questions [9]. A useful concept to broach a discussion about goals of care in the setting of a serious illness is to "hope for the best and plan for the worst" [10]. Discussions about goals of care take into account what the patient values in his or her life. These values provide direction in creating a care plan that integrates the patient's medical condition, hopes and worries about the future, and involvement of family and/or close friends in knowing a patient's priorities and wishes. The Conversation Project founded by the Institute for Healthcare Improvement has a starter kit to guide patients and families to think about how to have these difficult conversations (www.theconversationproject.org).

To actualize the patient's values while "planning for the worst," advanced care planning is addressed in different forms. As illustrated in the case scenario below, a patient may value interacting with his or her family as an important goal, and may forgo prolonged mechanical ventilation that would require sedation. A durable power of attorney for health care, or health care proxy, can be assigned to someone who can best advocate what the patient would want in a particular circumstance should the patient become incapacitated to make medical decisions. A living will and 5-Wishes (www.agingwithdignity.org) provide more specific details including life-sustaining therapy. Some U.S. states use a Physician Order for Life-Sustaining Treatments signed by a physician that stipulates the conditions for initiating cardiopulmonary resuscitation, circumstances when patients should be hospitalized, and other supportive treatments like feeding tubes and antibiotics. The optimal time to begin these series of conversation about advanced care planning occurs early in the disease trajectory when the patient still has decision making capacity and can vocalize his or her values and preferences.

Patients with BPD may have vacillating preferences that reflect their changing emotional state. They may ask for expertise advice, yet at the same time reject offers for help. Behaviors such as being demanding or aggressive, refusing to participate in care, or expressing feelings of helplessness may lead clinicians to be uncertain in how to provide compassionate care. For patients who are unable to commit to or willing to discuss advanced care planning and/or exhibit challenging behaviors, mental health clinicians can take a step back and refocus their efforts on better understanding the patient's experience of being seriously ill. The exploration of a sick person's experience can reveal hopes and worries, priorities, understanding of prognosis, and affective response to being ill.

Case – Ms. J

Ms. J, a 70-year-old female with advanced non-small cell lung cancer, was admitted to the hospital for evaluation of syncope and chest pain. Prior to being diagnosed with lung cancer five years ago, Ms. J had resigned from her job as an accountant after multiple leaves of absence during the time of her divorce from her second husband. She had a 35-year-old son and a 30-year-old daughter whom she did not speak. She stated that her daughter had expressed no interest in her care. She had a history of heavy alcohol use in her first marriage. She was prescribed lithium early in her life, but she did not remember why. Ms. J had a history of self-injurious behavior, usually cutting her wrist with a razor or burning her forearm with cigarettes. In addition, when she and her second husband were on the verge of separating, she had one incident of overdosing on diphenhydramine.

On admission, her chief complaint was a two-day history of lightheadedness that started after she stopped eating, related to her anger over multiple unsuccessful attempts to contact her daughter. Ms. J was a thin, short, Caucasian woman with dyed blonde hair who was well dressed and hyperverbal with some psychomotor agitation. When asked about her mood, she smiled and stated that she was feeling the best she had felt in days. She was perseverative about her son's involvement in her care, speaking tearfully about his sacrifices for her.

During the hospitalization, Ms. J was approached by a nurse who placed a peripheral intravenous line. Ms. J complimented the nurse before she left, telling her she hardly felt the intravenous line being placed. The nurse later returned to place the telemetry monitor at which time Ms. J became agitated and told her that she had no idea what she was doing. Shortly thereafter, Ms. J complained of diffuse body pain and demanded to speak with the physician. She told the physician that she had been suffering from significant pain and did not know how she could continue living. Palliative care was consulted after she expressed feelings of helplessness and stated she had no support to make important decisions.

The palliative care team was faced with the following questions:

1.   What therapeutic approach should the team use to engage with Ms. J?

Ms. J experienced both physical and emotional distress. By exploring what factors she believed were contributing to her distress and addressing her concerns in a clear, direct way, the palliative care team validated her suffering. The team should be empathic, while avoiding excess identification/enmeshment with her through monitoring the feelings and countertransference in the clinical encounters.

2.   What goals should be delineated for Ms. J's care?

The primary team should assess Ms. J's understanding of her medical problems. This understanding would lead to conversations about her values and life goals, permitting the team to be involved in a shared-decision making process that respected her preferences and values. By identifying tensions in her relationships with her children, Ms. J could work toward reconciliation. The palliative care team also would be helpful in symptom control including providing appropriate pain management.

Ms. J told the palliative care team that after undergoing the last series of chemotherapy and radiation she began to feel weaker and hopeless, wondering if there was a point at which she should continue treatment given her physical deterioration and poor quality of life. She also lacked purpose and meaning in her life because she felt abandoned by those who were closest to her. While she was supported by her son, she began feeling like a burden to him since he had become a new father. She also lamented the rupture in her relationship with her daughter and desired to reconcile the relationship. She feared dying alone and did not want to live in pain. Because existential therapeutic interventions in the end-of-life care continue to receive increasing consideration, the search for meaning (grounded in Viktor Frankl's writings) has become an important resource for coping with emotional and existential suffering as one nears death [11]. This may be of significant importance particularly in patients with personality pathology. In our case, Ms. J and the palliative care physician discussed how her fears of abandonment and dying alone would abate if she repaired her relationship with her daughter and addressed the feelings of guilt and shame related to this fragile relationship.

Ms. J's medical condition continued to decline during her hospitalization, as her lung cancer metastasized to her liver and brain. She declined to pursue further treatment and instead focused on reconciling with her daughter. She planned to spend more time with her new grandchild. She desired to remain independent and did not want to spend her remaining days in the medical setting. Upon discussing with her oncologist the high probability that she would not be able to make further decisions for herself given the brain metastasis, she identified her son as the surrogate decision maker. Ms. J was discharged home with hospice care and died four weeks later. The palliative care team then met with Ms. J's children to provide grief counseling and validate their contributions to her care.

KEY POINTS: PALLIATIVE AND END-OF-LIFE CARE

- Palliative care targets symptom management, addresses stress associated with serious disease, and engages patients in advanced planning and shared decision making.
- Palliative care specialists and psychiatrists share the goals of addressing patients' concerns about their medical problems, facilitating insight into clinical scenarios and sense of meaning, and identifying priorities for the patients using a multidisciplinary approach.
- Patients with BPD who face serious medical illness may further demonstrate urgent care seeking behaviors, compromise their relationships with their surroundings, and amplify maladaptive coping mechanisms.
- Geriatric patients with BPD with terminal illness and angst associated with end-of-life care may be served by palliative care specialists for self-advocacy, addressing quality of life, enhancement of relationships, identifying goals of care, and assisting with the assignment of surrogate decision makers or healthcare proxy.

REFERENCES

[1]   Ferris FD, Balfour HM, Bowen K, et al. *A model to guide hospice palliative care: based on national principles and norms of practice.* Ottawa: Canadian Hospice Palliative Care Association; 2002.
[2]   von Gunten CF. Evolution and effectiveness of palliative care. *Am J Geriatr Psychiatry.* 2012; 20(4): 291-297.

[3] El-Jawahri A, Greer JA, Temel JS. Does palliative care improve outcomes for patients with incurable illness? A review of the evidence. *J Support Oncol.* 2011; 9(3): 87-94.

[4] Fairman N, Irwin SA. Palliative care psychiatry: update on an emerging dimension of psychiatric practice. *Curr Psychiatry Rep.* 2013; 15(7): 374.

[5] Hill R. End of life care for the patient with borderline personality disorder. *J Hosp Palliat Nurs.* 2005; 7(3): 150-161.

[6] Steinhauser KE, Christakis NA, Clipp EC, McNeilly M, McIntyre L, Tulsky JA. Factors considered important at the end of life by patients, family, physicians, and other care providers. *JAMA.* 2000; 284(19): 2476-2482.

[7] Block SD. Psychological issues in end-of-life care. *J Palliat Med.* 2006; 9(3): 751-772.

[8] Lacy TJ, Higgins MJ. Integrated medical-psychiatric care of a dying borderline patient: a case of dynamically informed "practical psychotherapy". *J Am Acad Psychoanal Dyn Psychiatry.* 2005; 33(4): 619-636.

[9] Goodlin SJ, Quill TE, Arnold RM. Communication and decision-making about prognosis in heart failure care. *J Card Fail.* 2008; 14(2): 106-113.

[10] Back AL, Arnold RM, Quill TE. Hope for the best, and prepare for the worst. *Ann Intern Med.* 2003; 138(5): 439-443.

[11] Breitbart W, Poppito S, Rosenfeld B, et al. Pilot randomized controlled trial of individual meaning-centered psychotherapy for patients with advanced cancer. *J Clin Oncol.* 2012; 30(12): 1304-1309.

SECTION IV

NEW DEVELOPMENTS AND FUTURE DIRECTIONS

In: Borderline Personality Disorder in Older Adults
Editors: A. Hategan, J. A. Bourgeois, G. L. Xiong

ISBN: 978-1-63482-221-3
© 2015 Nova Science Publishers, Inc.

Chapter 14

GERIATRIC BORDERLINE PERSONALITY DISORDER IN THE ERA OF THE DSM-5 AND ICD-11

Liesel-Ann Meusel[1], PhD, Margaret McKinnon[2], PhD, CPsych and Peter J. Bieling[3,], PhD, CPsych*

[1]Rotman Research Institute, Baycrest, Toronto, ON, Canada
[2]St. Joseph's Healthcare Hamilton, Homewood Research Institute,
and McMaster University, Hamilton, ON, Canada
[3]St. Joseph's Healthcare Hamilton and McMaster University,
Hamilton, ON, Canada

The development of a valid and reliable assessment tool for personality disorders has the potential to influence significantly treatment, management, and quality of life for individuals with personality difficulties. Here, we review briefly the current diagnostic criteria and classification of borderline personality disorder (BPD), with a focus on BPD in the recently released 5th edition of the Diagnostic and Statistical Manual for Mental Disorders (DSM-5), and in the context of the DSM-5 alternate model of personality disorders. Personality disorder presentation in older adults will also be discussed. There is an urgent need for future editions of the DSM and the upcoming 11th revision of the International Classification of Disease (ICD-11) to include guidelines that reflect accurately how personality disorders evolve with age and within the context of other medical disorders associated with aging (e.g., neurocognitive disorders/dementia).

INTRODUCTION

As evidenced by the scope of discussions presented thus far, BPD is a complex and heterogeneous cluster of symptoms that include characteristically emotional instability, low impulse control, unstable interpersonal relationships, and unstable self-image. This chapter will briefly review past, present, and future controversies around classification of BPD in the various iterations of the Diagnostic and Statistical Manual for Mental Disorders (DSM) and International Classification of Disease (ICD). Current developments and future directions will

---
[*] Corresponding author: pbieling@stjosham.on.ca.

also be discussed, where it is critical that upcoming editions of the DSM and ICD include enhanced guidelines that will aid clinicians with the diagnosis of BPD in older adults.

BORDERLINE PERSONALITY DISORDER IN THE ERA OF THE DSM-5

The categorical approach to personality disorder diagnosis first implemented by the DSM-III [1] has theoretical and pragmatic limitations. Over the years, clinicians and researchers have advocated for a shift away from the categorical approach, which considers personality disorders to be qualitatively distinct clinical syndromes, in favor of a personality disorder diagnostic system based on a dimensional framework, where personality traits exist on a spectrum and personality disorders represent the extremes of these normal personality traits [2-4]. In the early stages of its planning and conceptualization, the DSM-5 [5] was expected to incorporate such a system as the primary diagnostic framework for personality disorders.

The impetus for change to the personality disorder diagnostic system in the DSM comes from several sources. There is frustration with the excessive diagnostic comorbidity that exists amongst the personality disorders in their current categorical classification, and with the overall lack of validity [6], low 10-year test-retest stability [7] and general lack of empirical support for many of the specific disorders and their diagnostic thresholds [8, 9]. There is also frustration with the high degree of heterogeneity that exists within a specific personality disorder diagnosis. In the case of BPD, the requirement that at least five of nine criteria need to be endorsed means the different combinations that can lead to a diagnosis are numerous. The model put forth by many as the basis on which to build the new diagnostic system was the Five Factor Model of personality, a dimensional model of normal personality structure with high construct validity, high 10-year test-retest stability, and volumes of empirical support [10-13] (Also see Chapter 2 for more details on the Five Factor Model).

The DSM-5 personality disorder workgroup made significant progress developing an alternative, dimensional model of personality disorder [14] that aligned well with the previous, categorical model [15]. In this model, diagnosis of a personality disorder requires two determinations: an assessment of the level of impairment in personality functioning (Criterion A), and an evaluation of pathological personality traits (Criterion B). As detailed later in this section and using BPD as an example, Criterion A is meant to establish, across four domains (identity, self-direction, intimacy, and empathy), the overall degree of functional impairment and "clinically significant distress" caused by the maladaptive or extreme personality traits. Criterion B, on the other hand, attempts to characterize each individual's personality trait profile across five dimensions: negative affect/ emotional stability, detachment/ extraversion, disinhibition/conscientiousness, antagonism/ agreeableness, and psychoticism/lucidity. More generally, the basic tenets of what constitutes a personality disorder have not changed in this alternative model, and Criterion A and B above are rated in consideration of several factors: (1) personality functioning and personality trait expression are relatively inflexible and pervasive across a broad range of personal and

Table 14-1. Diagnostic Criteria for BPD in the DSM-5 (2013), and proposed ICD-11 Criteria for a general Personality Disorder Diagnosis (21)

DSM-5 (Alternative Model - BPD)	ICD-11 (Personality Disorders)
Criterion A: Moderate or greater impairment in personality functioning, manifested by characteristic difficulties in *two or more* of the following four areas: *Identity:* • unstable or poorly developed self-image • excessive self-criticism • chronic emptiness • dissociative states under stress *Intimacy:* • intense, unstable close relationships, marked by mistrust, neediness, and anxious preoccupation with real or imagined abandonment • close relationships often viewed in extremes of idealization and devaluation and alternating between overinvolvement and withdrawal *Self-direction:* • instability in goals, values, career plans, etc. *Empathy:* • compromised ability to recognize the emotional needs of others • interpersonal hypersensitivity • perceptions of others are selectively biased toward negative attributes or vulnerabilities **Criterion B:** *Four or more* of the following seven pathological personality traits, at least one of which must be (5) impulsivity, (6) risk taking, or (7) hostility: **Domain: Negative Affect** 1. Emotional lability 2. Anxiousness 3. Separation insecurity 4. Depressivity **Domain: Disinhibition** 5. Impulsivity 6. Risk taking **Domain: Antagonism** 7. Hostility	**Proposed Primary Classification: Severity** *No personality disorder* • no personality disturbance *Personality difficulty* • some personality problems in certain situations but not universally *Personality disorder* • definite, well-demarcated personality problems across a range of situations *Complex personality disorder* • definite personality problems usually covering several personality domains and across all situations *Severe personality disorder* • as for complex disorder with personality problems leading to significant risk to self or others **Proposed Secondary Classification: Personality Domains** **Domain 1 - Asocial/Schizoid** • isolation from others, social indifference, aloofness, introspection, reduced expression of affect, suspicion, and lack of empathy **Domain 2 - Dyssocial/Antisocial** • lack of regard for the needs of others and by aggression, irresponsibility, insensitivity or callousness, deceit, and egocentricity **Domain 3 - Obsessional/Anankastic** • over-conscientious behaviour, excessive orderliness, perfectionism, inflexibility, and cautiousness **Domain 4 - Anxious/Dependent** • anxiousness, lack of self-confidence, shyness, timidity, dependence on others, reluctance to make decisions **Domain 5 - Emotionally Unstable (borderline)** • lability of mood (emotional dysregulation), inconsistent negative affect, impulsiveness, tendency to self-loathing and self-harm, and antagonism

social situations (Criterion C); (2) personality profiles are relatively stable across time, and personality disorder onsets can usually be traced back to adolescence or early adulthood (Criterion D); and (3) these difficulties are not better accounted for by another disorder, by a medication or substance, or by development or cultural factors [5, 16].

Viewed critically, this new model has a solid conceptual basis and provides an efficient approach to assessment [17]; however, concerns about feasibility and ease of use in a clinical setting were identified by numerous individuals [18, 19]. Given the general lack of consensus across the field, and the priority assigned to maintaining continuity with current clinical practice, the categorical classification system of the DSM-IV was retained in the DSM-5 as the primary means of personality disorder assessment. To stimulate development and research into the DSM-5 alternative model of personality pathology, however, it was published as an emerging model for further study (referred to in DSM-5 as Section III, Emerging Measures and Models). Further updates and enhanced clarity surrounding the diagnosis of personality disorders should be expected in future revisions to the DSM-5.

Ongoing attempts to revise and refine personality disorder diagnosis are not limited to the DSM. The upcoming release, in 2017, of the 11th revision of the International Classification of Disease (ICD-11; 20), is expected to come with major changes to the classification of personality disorders. Proposed changes include an emphasis, for diagnosis, on severity of personality disturbance rather than the nature of the disturbance (which echoes Criterion A of the DSM-5 alternative model), with a secondary classification aimed at qualifying the nature of the disturbance on five trait domains (echoing Criterion B of the DSM-5 alternative model) [21, 22]. Table 14-1 details what is known about the proposed structure of the ICD-11 for personality disorder diagnosis. These changes to the ICD come in response to the same factors that are pushing the DSM towards a dimensional model of personality. Whether the ICD-11 dimensional personality disorder classification system will face similar criticisms to the DSM-5 proposals (too complex, too impractical) remains to be seen. Certainly, in theory, dimensional models have great utility, but in every day work clinicians require practical and efficient tools to gather and organize the information these systems demand.

Nonetheless, dimensional models hoped for in the DSM and still planned for in the ICD-11 have the potential to improve validity and reliability of personality disorder diagnosis. This is particularly true if clinicians, on a wide scale, begin using similar assessment tools. Information gleaned from such measures should also facilitate treatment planning, a useful advance for clinicians. For example, a DSM-IV or DSM-5 diagnosis of BPD conveys little information about a particular patient's spectrum of personality dysfunction, which limits the degree to which treatment considerations can be inferred from diagnosis alone. In contrast, a personality profile generated using a dimensional approach to assessment will convey more nuanced information about each patient, which can be used to identify potential barriers to treatment or good prognostic indicators, and guide tailored treatment recommendations

FUTURE TRENDS IN THE DEVELOPMENT OF DIAGNOSTIC CRITERIA FOR BORDERLINE PERSONALITY DISORDER IN OLDER ADULTS

For years, groups have been calling on the DSM and other diagnostic systems to create guidelines, differential diagnoses, specifiers, or alternate criteria centered on the assessment of personality disorder in geriatric populations [23-25]. Some have suggested a geriatric subclassification for personality disorders to increase validity and reliability [26], while others called for the use of age-neutral DSM-IV items only, as well as informant reports, for personality assessment in older adults [27]. All agreed that without added supports, the utility of the DSM and other diagnostic systems for our aging population is limited by low validity and reliability in this group.

As detailed elsewhere in this volume, many studies suggest that BPD, and personality dysfunction more generally, decreases in severity across middle-age [28-31]; however, it is also accepted that a subset of patients, usually those with more severe personality dysfunction, continue to experience difficulties into senescence [31], with one meta-analysis estimating a 10% prevalence rate for personality disorders in older adults [32].

There is also evidence to show that the expression of maladaptive personality traits changes with increasing age [27], which calls into question whether the current DSM personality disorder criteria are adequately capturing the evolution of personality disorder expression as people age, and especially in older adults. For example, in the context of BPD, one study found that older adults with BPD were less likely to endorse what are considered to be the characteristic BPD symptoms: impulsivity, self-harm, substance use, and affective instability, but more likely to endorse feelings of chronic emptiness and report greater social impairment than their younger counterparts [33]. Differential endorsement of certain DSM personality disorder criteria in younger versus older adults, suggestive of a measurement bias across age groups, has been noted elsewhere [34], and some suggest that as many as one third of DSM-IV Axis II criteria (which were used in the former classification system to record personality pathologies but removed from the DSM-5 system) were inappropriate for use with older adults [27, 35]. Overall, these results are suggestive of a complex, dynamic pattern in which the early behavioral expression of BPD produces a stress-generating environment that has important intrapersonal and interpersonal costs as a person ages. But these are speculative observations, clouded by classification and instrumentation issues which require resolution.

Because of the conceptual and practical limitations described, personality disorders in older adults often go undetected [35, 36]. This underscores the need for even limited basic guidelines in the DSM or ICD to help clinicians navigate the diagnosis of geriatric BPD more consistently and reliably. For example, information and guidance within the DSM on the differential diagnosis of BPD from incipient vascular, metabolic, and neurodegenerative processes like frontotemporal neurocognitive disorder or Alzheimer's disease would be useful, where the onset of personality changes, including increased impulsivity, extreme mood lability, and difficulties maintaining norms of interpersonal interactions may be confused with personality disorder traits. It would also be helpful to publish additional criteria within each personality diagnosis to exemplify the characteristics of that diagnosis as expressed in older adults. As reviewed in this chapter, dimensional models of personality disorders, with continued refinement and careful attention to measurement, have the potential to improve the validity and reliability of personality disorder diagnosis in future editions of the DSM and ICD [37].

KEY POINTS: GERIATRIC BORDERLINE PERSONALITY DISORDER IN THE ERA OF THE DSM-5 AND ICD-11

- Accurate and timely diagnosis of personality pathology has the potential to be of great benefit to older adults with BPD, and those with personality dysfunction more generally.
- Proper diagnosis has implications for treatment facilitation, behavioral management, and, more broadly, quality of life for those coping with personality dysfunction.
- Dimensional models, coupled with reliable and valid assessment tools, have the potential to enhance greatly recognition and treatment of BPD. Dimensional models may result in a much better paradigm for studying both overt and subtle changes that occur in BPD as individuals age.

REFERENCES

[1]   American Psychiatric Association. *Diagnostic and Statistical Manual of Mental Disorders.* 3rd ed. Washington, DC: American Psychiatric Press, Inc., 1980.
[2]   Costa PT Jr, McCrae RR. Bridging the gap with the five-factor model. *Personal Disord.* 2010; 1: 127-130.
[3]   Widiger TA, Trull TJ. Plate tectonics in the classification of personality disorder: Shifting to a dimensional model. *Am Psychol.* 2007; 62: 71-83.
[4]   Widiger TA, Simonsen E. Alternative dimensional models of personality disorder: finding a common ground. *J Pers Disord.* 2005; 19(2): 110-130.
[5]   American Psychiatric Association. *Diagnostic and Statistical Manual of Mental Disorders.* 5th ed. Arlington, VA: American Psychiatric Publishing, 2013.
[6]   Kendell R, Jablensky A. Distinguishing between the validity and utility of psychiatric diagnoses. *Am J Psychiatry.* 2003; 160: 4-12.
[7]   Hopwood CJ, Morey LC, Donnellan MB, et al. Ten-year rank-order stability of personality traits and disorders in a clinical sample. *J Pers.* 2012; 81: 335-344.
[8]   Krueger RF, Eaton, N. Personality traits and the classification of mental disorders: Toward a more complete integration in DSM-5 and an empirical model of psychopathology. *Personal Disord.* 2010; 1: 97-118.
[9]   Balsis S, Lowmaster S, Cooper LD, Benge JF. Personality disorder diagnostic thresholds correspond to different levels of latent pathology. *J Pers Disord.* 2011; 25(1): 115-127.
[10] Costa PT Jr, McCrae RR. *The NEO Personality Inventory.* Odessa, FL: Psychological Assessment Resources; 1985.
[11] Costa PT, Jr., McCrae RR. Revised NEO Personality Inventory (NEO-PI-R) and NEO Five-Factor Inventory (NEO-FFI) manual. Odessa, *FL: Psychological Assessment Resources.* 1992.
[12] McCrae RR, Costa PT. Validation of the five-factor model of personality across instruments and observers. *Journal of Personality and Social Psychology.* 1987; 52(1): 81-90.

[13] Costa PT, Jr., McCrae RR. Personality disorders and the five-factor model of personality. *J Pers Disord.* 1990; 4(4): 362-371.

[14] Skodol AE. Personality disorders in DSM-5. *Annu Rev Clin Psychol.* 2012; 8: 317-344.

[15] Sellbom M, Sansone RA, Songer DA, Anderson JL. Convergence between DSM-5 Section II and Section III diagnostic criteria for borderline personality disorder. *Aust N Z J Psychiatry.* 2014; 48(4): 325-332.

[16] American Psychiatric Association. Diagnostic and Statistical Manual of Mental Disorders (4th ed.). Washington, DC: American Psychiatric Publishing, 1994.

[17] Skodol AE, Krueger RF, Bender DS, et al. Personality disorders in DSM-5 Section III. *Personal Disord.* 2013; 11(2): 187–188.

[18] Clarkin JF, Huprich SK. Do DSM-5 personality disorder proposals meet criteria for clinical utility? *J Pers Disord.* 2011; 25(2):192-205.

[19] Zimmerman M. A critique of the proposed prototype rating system for personality disorders in DSM-5. *J Pers Disord.* 2011; 25(2): 206-221.

[20] World Health Organization. The ICD-11 Classification of Mental and Behavioural Disorders: Clinical Descriptions and Diagnostic Guidelines. Geneva, CH, 2017 (expected release). http://www.who.int/classifications/icd/revision/en/. Accessed January, 10, 2015.

[21] Tyrer P, Crawford M, Mulder R, et al. The rationale for the reclassification of personality disorder in the 11th revision of the international classification of diseases (ICD-11). *Personal Ment Health.* 2011; 5(4): 246-259.

[22] Tyrer P, Crawford M, Mulder R, et al. Reclassification of personality disorder. *Lancet.* 2011; 377(9780): 1814-1815.

[23] Oldham JM, Skodol AE. Personality and personality disorders, and the passage of time. *Am J Geriatr Psychiatry.* 2013; 21: 709-712.

[24] Kroessler D. Personality disorder in the elderly. *Psychiatric Services.* 1990; 41(12): 1325-1329.

[25] Balsis S, Segal DL, Donahue C. Revising the personality disorder diagnostic criteria for the Diagnostic and Statistical Manual of Mental Disorders–Fifth Edition (DSM-V): consider the later life context. *Am J Orthopsychiatry.* 2009; 79: 452-460.

[26] Agronin ME, Maletta G. Personality Disorders in Late Life: Understanding and Overcoming the Gap in Research. *Am J Geriatr Psychiatry.* 2000; 8(1): 4-18.

[27] Debast I, van Alphen SPJ, Rossi G, et al. Personality traits and personality disorders in late middle and old age: do they remain stable? A literature review. *Clin Gerontol.* 2014; 37(3): 253-271.

[28] Paris J, Zweig-Frank H. A 27-year follow-up of patients with borderline personality disorder. *Compr Psychiatry.* 2001; 42(6): 482-487.

[29] Zanarini MC, Frankenburg FR, Hennen J, Reich DB, Silk KR. Prediction of the 10-year course of borderline personality disorder. *Am J Psychiatry.* 2006; 163(5): 827-832.

[30] Zanarini MC, Frankenburg FR, Reich DB, Fitzmaurice G. Attainment and stability of sustained symptomatic remission and recovery among patients with borderline personality disorder and axis II comparison subjects: a 16-year prospective follow-up study. *Am J Psychiatry.* 2012; 169(5): 476-83.

[31] Ames A, Molinari V. Prevalence of personality disorders in community living elderly. *J Geriatric Psychiatry Neurol.* 1994; 7: 189-194.

[32] Abrams RC, Horowitz SV. Personality disorders after age 50: a meta-analysis. *J Pers Disord.* 1996; 10(3): 271-281.

[33] Morgan TA, Chelminski I, Young D, Dalrymple K, Zimmerman MJ. Differences between older and younger adults with borderline personality disorder on clinical presentation and impairment. *Psychiatry Res.* 2013; 47(10): 1507-1513.

[34] Balsis S, Woods CM, Gleason MEJ, Oltmanns TF. Overdiagnosis and underdiagnosis of personality disorders in older adults. *Am J Geriatr Psychiatry.* 2007; 15(9): 742-753.

[35] Segal DL, Hersen M, Van Hasselt VB, Silberman, CS, Roth L. Diagnosis and assessment of personality disorders in older adults: a critical review. *J Pers Disord.* 1996; 10(4): 384-399.

[36] Jeyasingam N, Jacob KS, Brodaty H. Personality disorders in geriatric inpatients in a tertiary hospital. *Australas Psychiatry.* 2014; 22(5): 458-460.

[37] Andrews G, Goldberg DP, Krueger RF, et al. Exploring the feasibility of a meta-structure for DSM-V and ICD-11: could it improve utility and validity? *Psychol Med.* 2009; 39(12): 1993-2000.

ISBN: 978-1-63482-221-3
© 2015 Nova Science Publishers, Inc.

Chapter 15

SYSTEMIC CHALLENGES AND STRATEGIES FOR INSTITUTIONAL SETTINGS

Caroline Giroux[1,], MD, Andrew M. Bein[2], PhD and Glen L. Xiong[3], MD, CMD*

[1]Assistant Clinical Professor and APSS Stockton Clinic Medical Director,
Site Director for Clerkship and Residents at APSS Stockton,
University of California at Davis, Sacramento, CA, US
[2]Professor, Division of Social Work,
California State University, Sacramento, CA, US
[3]Health SciencesAssociate Clinical Professor, Psychiatry Department of Psychiatry
and Behavioral Sciences, University of California, at Davis, Sacramento, CA, US

The high prevalence of patients with borderline personality combined with their specific comorbid conditions increase the likelihood of encountering them in various institutional settings. With aging, they become at higher risk of medical complications. To maximize therapeutic efficacy, treatment infrastructures should be prepared to respond to such needs. Some pejorative labels commonly used by clinicians can help identify challenges inherent to serving that population and approaches can be adjusted accordingly. Encouraging self-awareness of emotional responses, self-regulation and validation at the staff level will help model beneficial skills among the patients themselves. From a case scenario to illustrate the challenges, this chapter will address three contributing sets of factors (patient, clinician, and situation) in difficult encounters. Three corresponding levels of strategies are illustrated, from screening and education to supervision groups and team approach to resource management.

INTRODUCTION

Because of the significantly high prevalence of borderline personality disorder (BPD) among various treatment settings (6% in primary care, 10% in outpatient mental health and 20% among psychiatric inpatients) [1], early diagnosis and management can impact the

---
*Corresponding author: caroline.giroux@ucdmc.ucdavis.edu.

outcome, even among the geriatric population. As stated elsewhere in this book, the prevalence may decrease in older age group (e.g., age-associated "burnout" of certain features such as impulsivity) but some maladaptive characteristics can be exacerbated by the accumulation of various losses and iatrogenic injuries. This may create difficult clinical encounters, which are estimated to represent 15-30% of family physician visits [2].

Factors Contributing to Challenging Clinical Interactions

Contributing factors to difficult clinical encounters are regrouped in three categories: the patient, the clinician, and the situation.

Phenomenology: The Patient

A poor boundary definition plays a central role in the psychopathological expression of BPD. In most cases, there is a history of major trauma (e.g., emotional, physical, and/or sexual) followed by a component of invalidation from nurturing figures (which can be experienced as more traumatic than the abuse itself). Sexual abuse is a major boundary violation of the whole person, not just the body. If this violation occurs when the personality is still developing, it may lead to difficulties differentiating one's own emotional experiences, needs, self-image, and sets of beliefs from the external world. As a result, people with BPD appear unstable, a little bit like "emotional magnets", wanting to be either too close or too distant (maybe secondarily to hypersensitivity to abandonment), and self-destructive (often as attempts to dissociate or, conversely, to "feel" some emotional experience rather than an unpleasant "numbness"; this feature tends to decrease with age though). They also may have distorted perceptions of the world and themselves (e.g., bodily sensations, emotions). There is a female predominance in prevalence (75%) [3]. Having often suffered chronic trauma, across the lifespan she can present a combination of mood, anxiety, eating or substance-related disorders. Pain syndromes, gynecological conditions (e.g., often referable to the complications of sexual assault, multiple pregnancies, abortions, sexually transmitted diseases), and narcotic dependence are likely to be diagnosed across various specialties. A patient requesting multiple investigations or procedures (e.g., plastic surgery) can reveal body image issues or somatic manifestations. BPD was found to be specifically associated with insomnia in later middle-aged adults in the community [4].

Case – Ms. T

Ms. T, a 67-year-old woman with type-2 diabetes and congestive heart failure, was admitted to the medicine unit for exacerbation of congestive heart failure. Her hemoglobin A1C was concerning (12%) and she weighed 251 pounds (BMI: 42). She was cordial to the physicians during morning rounds but on some days was tense and refused vital sign measurement if done by a male nurse.

The hospitalist physician was astonished to hear the nursing staff complain that the patient was being very "difficult", "a whiner", who dismissed the medical student's patient explanations of her condition and treatments, expressing her great frustration to still have shortness of breath despite 5 days of treatment with diuretics. She asked about each of her pills before taking them. She did not follow fluid restrictions and frequently flushed her urine without saving it for output measurement. Nurses suspected that she was asking her youngest daughter to "sneak in" fast food and sodas for her. After those visits, Ms. T got very down, feeling "insignificant, rejected" but was rather irritable when her older daughter showed up (which "aggravated" her, just like some nurses). Staff characterized her as "entitled" for yelling at the nursing assistant for being slow in helping her to use the restroom.

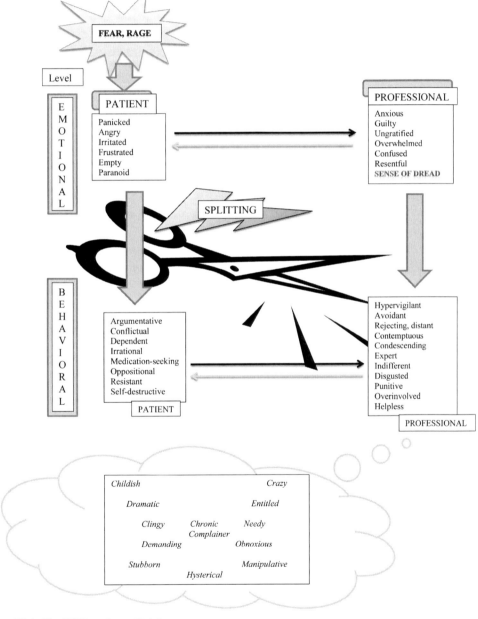

Figure 15-1. The BPD patient-clinician encounter.

This case scenario illustrating a "difficult, manipulative and entitled" patient also exemplifies patients frequently hospitalized for multiple exacerbations of a chronic medical problem. While the patient is getting treatment in a confined institution such as a hospital, her interpersonal tendency to idealize some of the clinicians and to devalue others can interfere with care delivery. This internal splitting might be projected so powerfully that the clinical team itself will enact it, sometimes at the patient's expense (See Figure 15-1).

Clinicians often feel "frustrated, ungratified, and guilty" [5], when treating these "demanding" patients. Figure 15-1 illustrates the feedback mechanisms of emotional and behavioral experiences triggered by powerful affects such as anger or fear. These lead to the use of pejorative labels (as seen in Figure 15-1, italic type), and should prompt a consideration of a diagnosis of BPD.

Patients with BPD struggle with emotion regulation [6]. Their behaviors and presentation may seem to be expected and justified due to disability and losses that occur in old age. However, their disappointment over what appears to some as trivial stimuli may turn into despair or rage. Externalizing hostility may be a defense against experiencing what many people with BPD frequently suffer: a profound sense of unworthiness and of not being validated.

The Clinician's Role

Every clinician brings a specific background, personality, and set of skills in each encounter. Through acknowledging our own internal processes, our task is to validate and accept the emotional experience of patients with BPD, while maintaining professional boundaries and assisting the patient in containing her or his emotional reactivity. The first step to facilitate greater therapeutic success in the clinical encounter is clinician self-awareness.

Observing and accepting rather than condemning what occurs internally – in this case resentment and negative thoughts – means validation of one's own emerging experience. This, in turn, will facilitate validation of the patient's suffering.

The ingredients of mindful observation and validation of internal experience are the rehabilitative components for persons struggling with BPD [7]. If clinicians are able to model affective non-reactivity and calmness, patients are more likely to feel heard and validated. Additionally, if we cultivate a compassionate approach vis-à-vis ourselves, we will model for patients the essence of taking care of oneself and "being a friend to one's self" [8]. As professionals, we engage in *mindful acceptance* of our own reactivity in the face of a patient's emotional dysregulation. Or, we dispassionately see those feelings and thoughts for what they are, and seek to kindly take care of ourselves and to develop a *skillful response* [9]. Acceptance does not imply approval nor does it suggest an apathetic, laissez-faire response. Similar to the way in which we want to address our patients, acceptance means a *non-reactive* acknowledgment of our internal experience or of circumstances we cannot change.

William Madsen discusses the importance of seeing the *relational* character of resistance embedded in helping relationships [10]. When people do not follow advice, seem displeased with their connections with clinicians, or skeptically challenge "expert" opinion, they are labeled as non-compliant. The remedy suggested is to acknowledge the reality of resistance by reframing it as "reluctance." Such a non-judgmental stance normalizes our struggles as clinicians and places us on a collaborative path, making us more likely to listen and be caring.

Deconstructing resistance (for instance, by noticing the rigidity of medical institutions) helps us become more empathic with our patients. We have to understand them through the lens of trying to get their needs met. Our acceptance of these dynamics helps validate their internal experience – a key to healing for patients with BPD [7].

There are boundaries regarding how complaints and emotions may be expressed. These boundaries, of course, vary among settings. While one-to-one in a therapist's office, emotional distress is permissible to a point; at the nursing station, emotional containment – with a compassionate tone – is quickly the primary aim. Agreeing on achievable goals is at the core of a patient-centered approach.

Institutional Challenges: Situational Factors

In addition to the hospital as an example of an institutional setting, assisted-living and skilled nursing facility is likely the largest "institution" that provides both housing and medical care for older adults. Traditionally, a serious mismatch has persisted between mental health needs and resources of nursing facilities [11]. Even an outpatient clinic is a form of institution, as it comes with policies, procedures and resource limitations that can be constraining towards a patient if excessive rigidity is exercised. Figure 15-2 illustrates the "matryoshka doll-like" configuration of the environmental factors.

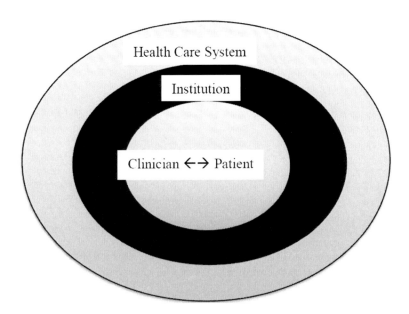

Figure 15-2. Examples of Categories of Environmental Factors.

Nevertheless, some of the obstacles or challenges stemming from the clash between a rigid institutional setting and an older adult with BPD can be alleviated, if not avoided.

Strategies

Vague, multiple or unexplained somatic symptoms, benzodiazepine dependence, polypharmacy, unpleasant countertransference should initiate screening for BPD and other comorbid conditions. Psychoeducation of patients about BPD and its recommended treatments is often neglected. It is fundamental to shape overall attitudes towards a better understanding of BPD. If we view the diagnosis as pejorative, we become reluctant to disclose it to the patient [3], which deprives her or him of important resources and of taking responsibility for their care. Participating in their diagnosis empowers the patients, which is of tremendous importance with a person having potentially suffered major trauma. Once the diagnosis of BPD has been explained, we should maintain a nonjudgmental, caring attitude towards the patient.

Lateral communication among multidisciplinary healthcare professionals in reassessment of interventions should be done on a regular basis, especially in settings of high acuity. For the medical-surgical hospital, a possible pragmatic solution would be to involve nurses during morning rounds and review the more challenging patients so that the physicians and nurses adopt a consistent approach with such patients. A proactive (rather than reactive) approach that could help prevent crises would consist of incorporating mindfulness exercises as a daily routine for staff and patients, helping patients define/consolidate boundaries and self-regulate in a healthy manner, for example, after a separation or change of clinician. Our firm, empathetic approach would be like an "institutional cast" for their developing and healing ego.

Apart from patient-centered approaches and techniques to increase the clinician's awareness and competency, structuring parameters such as access to educational material, setting and frequency of visits should be established. Some patients would benefit from shorter, more frequent visits, especially when the list of complaints is long or when it is during the evaluation process. Others prefer an agreed upon time.

Last but not least, these aspects should continue to be part of the management even beyond the date of discharge. Ensuring proper liaison through effective communication will consolidate compliance.

Figure 15-3 lists examples of multi-modal approaches at the patient, staff, and structural levels.

Case – Ms. T (Continued)

In order to avoid the "splitting" among team members, the senior psychiatry resident and nurse manager met to discuss the complex interpersonal dynamics and develop a consistent approach. Moreover, the inpatient team outlined basic expectations to Ms. T such as adhering to fluid restriction and participation in vital signs and urine output measurements. Extensive education and risk-benefit analysis was provided. The team elicited her thoughts about the dietary and fluid restrictions. Ms. T felt strongly that she should be allowed to eat anything but understood the consequences. The team respected her choice, as the patient may likely continue her dietary practice when she leaves the hospital. Also, the team stopped insisting on an extraordinarily rigid fluid restriction, and she started to regulate her fluid in a more practical manner that was reflective of her intake at home. Giving up an authoritarian or over-controlling attitude and replacing it by compassionate awareness ended up being fruitful by decreasing her resistance. A social worker was consulted to use motivational interviewing and teach stress-reduction techniques to Ms. T. Allowing the patient to make mistakes (within safe boundaries) made her accountable for her decisions. She felt rewarded, which ultimately improved her health outcomes.

In summary, early recognition of BPD can better prepare clinicians to plan effective treatment that engages the patient (e.g., more realistic dietary and fluid restrictions), make him or her accountable and reduce further medical complications.

Patients struggling with BPD may end up hospitalized in various medical specialty facilities. Hence, we have a central role in screening and initiating appropriate interventions. Moreover, institutions have the advantage of providing a transitional space where healing and learning can occur for patients who struggle with emotional dysregulation. Classes on BPD, expressing validation, teaching mindfulness and other stress-reducing strategies among staff and patients are essential. Just as important, the team should encourage accountability by asking these patients to take an active role in their treatment and healing process.

As clinicians, we would benefit from being aware of our sense of dread or other negative feelings (such as anger and frustration) and use self-reflection, supervision, mindfulness techniques and other therapies as needed [12]. Within safe boundaries, clinicians should strive to *meet people with patience and empathy* and recognize familiar labels that distance us from our patients. Tolerating uncertainty, trusting the patient's ability to grow and learn will also help us accept our own limits.

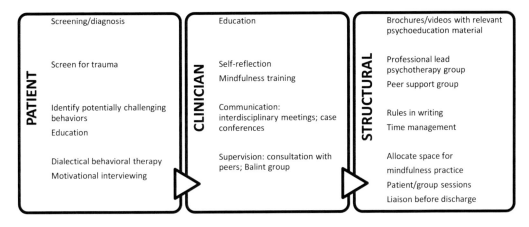

Figure 15-3. Institutional Approaches to Borderline Personality Disorder.

We should not underestimate the complexity of treating BPD in institutions. A clearer understanding of the multi-dimensional aspects sets the stage for a more effective intervention, no matter in which facility the patient receives care.

KEY POINTS: SYSTEMIC CHALLENGES AND STRATEGIES FOR INSTITUTIONAL SETTINGS

- BPD is common in treatment settings and early identification can positively affect treatment outcomes.

- Patients with BPD can evoke strong emotional reactivity from clinicians. During difficult encounters, we have to examine the complex dynamics between the variables at the patient, clinician, and institutional levels.
- A multi-leveled approach within institutions targeting these 3 sets of factors is likely to optimize recovery or help achieve stabilization and decrease professional exhaustion.
- Education, training, and self-care are key aspects leading to a more empathetic, validating attitude.
- Communication among team members is essential to ensure consistency and structure.
- The multidisciplinary treatment plan should take into account the living environment after discharge (home versus nursing facility).

REFERENCES

[1]   American Psychiatric Association. Diagnostic and Statistical Manual of Mental Disorders. 5th ed. Arlington, VA: American Psychiatric Publishing, 2013; 665.

[2]   Cannarella Lorenzetti R, Jacques CH, Donovan C, Cottrell S, Buck J. Managing difficult encounters: Understanding physician, patient, and situational factors. *Am Fam Physician.* 2013; 87(6): 419-425.

[3]   Gunderson JG. Borderline personality disorder. *N Engl J Med.* 2011; 364: 2037-2042.

[4]   Oltmanns JR, Weinstein Y, Oltmanns TF. Borderline personality pathology and insomnia symptoms in community-dwelling older adults. *Personal Ment Health.* 2014; 8(3): 178-187.

[5]   Bair MJ. Patient encounters of a difficult kind. *J Gen Intern Med.* 2014; 29(8): 1083-1084.

[6]   Linehan MM. *Skills Training Manual for Treating Borderline Personality Disorder.* New York, NY: Guilford, 1993.

[7]   Bein A. Dialectical behavior therapy for wellness and recovery: Interventions and activities for diverse client needs. Hoboken, NJ: Wiley, 2014.

[8]   Siegel DJ. *Mindsight: The new science of personal transformation.* New York, NY: Bantam, 2010.

[9]   Kabat-Zinn J. *Full catastrophe living: Using the wisdom of your body and mind to face stress, pain, and illness.* New York, NY: Dell, 1990.

[10] Madsen WC. Collaborative therapy with multi-stressed families. 2nd ed. New York, NY: Guilford Press, 2007

[11] Streim JE. Psychiatric problems in nursing homes. In: Sheikh JI, 1st ed. *Treating the Elderly.* 1st ed. San Francisco, CA: Jossey-Bass Inc., 1996, 195-219.

[12] Sanyer O, Fortenberry K. Using mindfulness techniques to improve difficult clinical encounters. *Am Fam Physician.* 2013; 87(6): 402.

In: Borderline Personality Disorder in Older Adults   ISBN: 978-1-63482-221-3
Editors: A. Hategan, J. A. Bourgeois, G. L. Xiong   © 2015 Nova Science Publishers, Inc.

Chapter 16

CONSIDERATIONS FOR ACCOUNTABLE CARE ORGANIZATIONS AND MEDICAL HOMES

Shannon Suo[1,], MD and Sid Stacey[2], MHSc*
[1]Associate Clinical Professor, University of California, at Davis,
Department of Psychiatry and Behavioral Sciences,
Sacramento, CA, US
[2]Assistant Professor (PT) and Director of Administration,
Department of Psychiatry and Behavioural Neurosciences,
Faculty of Health Sciences, McMaster University,
Hamilton, ON, Canada

This is an exciting time for healthcare delivery worldwide. We have a burgeoning science that is helping us understand the origins of disease and improve treatment in our geriatric patients. This comes at a time of immense change in payment and delivery systems that is important for mental health clinicians to understand. This chapter provides a summary of the recent legal and administrative initiatives in the U.S. referable to the Affordable Care Act of great importance in providing clinical care to geriatric patients, particularly those diagnosed with borderline personality disorder (BPD), with an emphasis on the provision of psychiatric services in the U.S. We also include a discussion of institutional systems of care for older patients in the Canadian healthcare system both for international comparison and to illustrate other creative approaches to the worldwide growing challenges in care delivery in institutional settings.

INTRODUCTION

In the U.S. in 2011, 17.7% of the gross domestic product (GDP) was spent on healthcare, compared with no more than 11.9% in any other industrialized country [1]. This helps to understand the need for recent initiatives in health care reform which hope to broaden access, contain costs, and focus on health benefits to the population at large. By contrast, we include

* Corresponding author: shannon.suo@ucdmc.ucdavis.edu.

a detailed discussion of how the health care delivery system is organized in Canada, to illustrate an alternative model.

As the changes in the U.S. system in the last 5 years are an abrupt, discontinuous change from the previous model, we will focus the majority of this chapter on the implications of the changes in the U.S. system for clinicians treating geriatric patients in institutional settings.

HEALTH CARE REFORM

The Patient Protection and Affordable Care Act of 2010, more commonly referred to as the Affordable Care Act/ACA, began to be implemented in January, 2014. There are many issues that are beyond the scope of this chapter to discuss; it is not the intent of this chapter to discuss the merits or the rationale behind the ACA, nor the individual differences of implementation by states, but rather to provide an overview of the Act and related legislation as it impacts the care of geriatric patients with BPD.

The ACA is being implemented at a time of reform of the medical system from other quarters. The Paul Wellstone and Pete Domenici Mental Health Parity and Addiction Equality Act of 2008 (MHPAEA) requires parity between mental health/substance use disorder benefits and medical-surgical benefits with respect to financial requirements and treatment limitations. The MHPAEA did not apply to Medicaid, Medicare, or small employer plans but the ACA requires elements of parity under the "essential health benefits" and amended the MHPAEA to apply to individual health insurance, such as those plans obtained through the state health exchanges. In January 2013, CMS (Centers for Medicare and Medicaid Services) issued expectations of Medicaid managed care plans to conform with the most basic of the parity requirements (i.e., co-pay, deductible limits, quantitative/non-quantitative therapy limits, out-of-network coverage, and medical necessity determinations) [2]. It is important to note that when state coverage or parity laws are *more* inclusive/restrictive, state law takes precedence over either the ACA or MHPAEA. For example, in California, the cutoff for eligibility for Medicaid is an annual income less than 138% of the federal poverty limit and many states broaden the definition of "mental disorders" to include all those in the most recent edition of the Diagnostic and Statistical Manual of Mental Disorders (DSM). The ACA also led to the definition of essential health benefits to include mental health and substance use disorder services.

To understand how the ACA impacts the psychiatric care of patients, we provide an overview of the changes brought about by the ACA. The ACA expanded coverage of individuals in two major ways: Medicaid expansion and the establishment of Health Insurance Exchanges. Geriatric patients, as defined by age 65 years and over will largely be covered by Medicare in the U.S. and are generally not included in expanded coverage unless ineligible for Medicare and obtaining coverage through the state exchange or Medicaid.

Medicaid

In the U.S., Medicaid is generally a government sponsored health insurance for eligible citizens with low income. The U.S. Supreme Court ruled that expansion of Medicaid was optional, so (as of this writing) 21 states have elected to *not* expand coverage for Medicaid [3]. For those states (and the District of Columbia) who have expanded Medicaid, uninsured individuals/families whose income falls below 133% of the federal poverty level are required to enroll unless exempted. The Medicaid plans themselves are state-dependent, but must offer, at a minimum, "Essential Health Benefits," including coverage for mental health and substance use disorders. The scope of the benefits offered by the state Medicaid plan must be "substantially equal to" the scope of benefits offered by a "benchmark plan" (See Figure 16-1 for a Benchmark Plan definition; 4). These requirements set a minimum amount of services available to recipients of Medicaid. "Medically frail" (including people with "disabling mental disorders") and "dual-eligibles" (eligible/receiving Medicaid and Medicare) are exempt from enrollment in the benchmark plans and may remain on "traditional" or fee-for-service Medicaid.

Health Care Exchanges

The state-based health care exchanges, or Health Insurance Marketplace, allow individuals to obtain private insurance for themselves or their families at rates comparable to those negotiated by larger companies. Applicants whose income is 133-400% of the federal poverty limit are eligible for sliding scale premium assistance (subsidy) by the federal government, but all income levels are able to purchase. Similar to employer-based insurance, plans obtained through the Marketplace have open enrollment between November 15 of the year prior to February 15 of the plan year, unless qualifying events occur. The ACA also prevents discrimination against patients for pre-existing conditions in determination of coverage and eliminates lifetime treatment limitations/caps on coverage. Figure 16-2 provides an example of insurance costs through California's Marketplace [4, 5]. Patients insured through Marketplace plans will benefit from the MHPAEA and ACA the most. Mental health and substance use disorders are essential health benefits, and subject to parity legislation. Therapeutic modalities previously difficult to have authorized or reimbursed, such as dialectical behavioral therapy, should be covered.

Federal Employees Health Benefit Plan

State Employee Health Benefit Coverage

The largest commercial (non-Medicaid) HMO plan in the state

Other Secretary-approved coverage, including those actuarially equivalent to one of the 3 above

---

Figure 16-1. Benchmark Plan Definition [4].

66 y/o* individual with an annual income of $16,105 (139% federal poverty level), tax credit for premium of $614-791/month:

Bronze (average 60% health plan coverage**): $1/month
Silver (70%**): $25-510***
Gold (80%**): $195-870***
Platinum (90%**): $293-1131***

Same person, annual income of $46,670 (400% FPL), tax credit for premium of $466/month:

Bronze: $150-247***
Silver: $350-835***
Gold: $250-1195***
Platinum: $619-1457***

* Prices applicable for age 62+
** Insured individuals/families are responsible for the remainder of the costs, typically in the form of co-pays, deductibles, etc.
*** Differences in costs within tiers are attributable to differences in costs of different plans/providers.

Figure 16-2. Example of Insurance Costs through California's Marketplace [4, 5].

Therefore, providers and patients must remain vigilant for inconsistent application of co-pays, deductibles, authorization/medical utilization review, and quantitative/non-quantitative treatment limitations. Violations of this law should be brought to the attention of the state insurance commissioner if the plan does not respond to reasonable attempts to appeal.

Medicare

Medicare is U.S. federally operated health insurance for people 65 years or older, younger people with selected disability, and those with end-stage kidney disease. The MHPAEA does *not* apply to Medicare. The ACA has minimal effects on Medicare. Patients are eligible for preventive services, including an annual "Wellness visit," without having to pay a deductible or co-pay. This simple change may provide an opportunity for geriatric patients, who commonly have medical comorbidities, to see a primary care provider on at least an annual basis at no cost (previously charged a 20% co-pay). The ACA also gradually closes the "donut hole" for prescription drug coverage until 2020, allowing patients to obtain their Medicare Part D-covered prescriptions at a gradually decreasing cost until it reaches the current non-donut hole cost of 25%.

The ACA mandates the implementation of a Medicare prospective payment system (PPS) for Federally Qualified Health Centers (FQHCs) beginning October 1, 2014. This replaces the Medicare Part B traditional fee-for-service structure for FQHCs only. From October 1, 2014 to December 31, 2015 the PPS rate is $158.85 multiplied by the geographic adjustment factor for the FQHC (the PPS is determined annually) [6]. However, FQHCs can bill for separate visits when a mental health visit occurs on the same day as a medical visit. The rate is also increased by 34% for new patients (not seen by the FQHC or off-site authorized "satellite" clinic of the FQHC within 3 years) or for a comprehensive initial Medicare visit or an annual wellness visit. Note that patients seen by a mental health provider for the first time are not considered new patients if they have been seen by another provider of the FQHC (even in another specialty) within 3 years.

ACCOUNTABLE CARE ORGANIZATIONS

The Accountable Care Organizations (ACOs) are entities that accept accountability for the cost and quality of care provided to a defined population and are comprised of a broad continuum of providers such as hospitals, medical homes, physician practices, primary care, community care, and home care services [7]. The primary objectives of ACOs are to increase quality of care, reduce costs and enhance population health and are premised on a new healthcare delivery model which shifts the focus from providers and their inputs to patients and outcomes. Although there has been considerable interest in ACOs in the U.S., many jurisdictions throughout the world are moving forward with implementing these new organizational structures. There are approximately 700 ACOs in the U.S. covering 6.1% of the national population [8]. The United Kingdom has recently implemented an accountable care program called Integrated Care Pioneers with the objective to enhance health outcomes and strengthen patient-centered health care [8]. The Agency for Integrated Care in Singapore launched the Agency for Integrated Care to reform long-term care delivery for geriatric patients with chronic conditions [8]. Outcomes reported include a 40% reduction in readmission rates and a 50% reduction in emergency department visits amongst its enrollees. The Agency for Integrated Care is launching new initiatives in mental health and social care. Canada, with its single-payer health system, has introduced regional integrated delivery systems that support population health, outcome measurement and coordinated delivery. Ontario in particular, Canada's largest province, has introduced Local Health Integrated Networks (LHINs) to better coordinate and integrate care delivery [9]. Behavioural Supports Ontario works at the local level to provide mentorship and support capacity for front line staff and mobile outreach to support geriatric patients and caregivers in the community when in crisis.

ACOs have important implications for geriatric patients with a diagnosis of BPD [10]. The National Survey of Accountable Care Organizations reports that ACOs with a community health center are more likely to integrate behavioral health into primary care (28% vs. 8%). This emphasis on care coordination and patient-centered delivery systems appears to influence care provided to geriatric patients with chronic conditions such as BPD. As ACOs continue to evolve, health systems need to monitor access and outcome measures for geriatric patients with BPD.

MEDICAL HOMES

The U.S. Agency for Healthcare Research and Quality defines the Patient Centered Medical Home as an organizational construct that provides comprehensive health care, including mental health care needs, prevention, acute and chronic care [11]. The primary care provider is responsible for coordination of all of the patient's care across inpatient, outpatient, and all specialists. If the medical home is unable to provide the specialty care directly, it is responsible for obtaining the care within a defined period of time (often contractually or state-determined), which is also affected by acuity. This model provides the opportunity for mental health specialists to work within the primary care office, consult with the primary care provider, or remain in a traditional separate location [12]. Working with primary care may require some cultural changes for mental health providers depending on their role with the medical home: more flexible availability for consultation, not seeing patients and providing consultation based on structured or "curbside" reports, sharing of information on a more proactive basis.

However, given the tendencies of patients with BPD to split and the frequency and severity of medical comorbidities that geriatric patients have, increased coordination between providers should be beneficial to the entire team.

The Medical Home model is not limited to primary care, and U.S. Substance Abuse and Mental Health Service Administration - Health Resources and Services Administration (SAMHSA-HRSA) Center for Integrated Solutions issued a paper in 2012 supporting a Behavioral Health-based medical home that is based in mental health rather than a primary care setting. These "behavioral health homes" maintain the core identity of coordination and assurance of care, but meet the patient where they are more frequently encountered - the mental health setting.

Behavioral health homes require increased resources and/or relationships to assure medical care provision, but ensure that the mental health needs of the patient are more likely to be met [13]. In January 2014, the U.S. Joint Commission began issuing Behavioral Health Home Certification to organizations that are able to meet this higher standard. Evidence supports increased integration and coordination of care that is likely to positively impact geriatric patients with BPD and healthcare delivery is changing to adapt to this new model [14].

KEY POINTS: CONSIDERATIONS FOR ACCOUNTABLE CARE ORGANIZATIONS AND MEDICAL HOMES

- Traditional health delivery systems have not effectively addressed the health needs of the older adults with chronic conditions, particularly mental illness.
- In the U.S. health care system, the Affordable Care Act of 2010 has led to the creative development of new care delivery systems focusing on treatment access, clinical outcomes, and population health. Clinicians caring for geriatric patients with BPD will likely be interfacing with new systems of care delivery for these patients in the U.S.
- ACOs, medical homes, and integrated/collaborative care provide alternatives to the traditional medical and mental health system worldwide that offer opportunities to improve care to the vulnerable population of geriatric patients with BPD.

REFERENCES

[1]   Health at a Glance 2013, OECD Indicators. OECD Publishing, 2013.

[2]   Letter to state Medicaid directors and state health officials. Centers for Medicare and Medicaid Services. http://www.medicaid.gov/Federal-Policy-Guidance/downloads/ SHO-13-001.pdf. Issued January 16, 2013. Accessed November 20, 2014.

[3]   Status of Sate Action on the Medicaid Expansion Decision. Kaiser Family Foundation. http://kff.org/health-reform/state-indicator/state-activity-around-expanding-medicaid-under-the-affordable-care-act/. Updated August, 28, 2014. Accessed November 20, 2014.

[4]   Benchmark Benefits. Medicaid.gov. http://www.medicaid.gov/Medicaid-CHIP-Program-Information/By-Topics/Benefits/Benchmark-Benefits.html. Accessed November 20, 2014.

[5]   The Covered California Shop and Compare Tool. Covered California Website. http://www.coveredca.com/shopandcompare/#calculator. Accessed November 20, 2014.

[6]   CMS Finalizes a Medicare Prospective Payment System for Federally Qualified Health Centers. CMS.gov website. http://www.cms.gov/ Center/Provider-Type/Federally-Qualified-Health-Centers-FQHC-Center.html. Issued May 2, 2104. Accessed November 20, 2014.

[7]   Shortell SM. Accountable Care: U.S. and Global Challenges and Lessons, Moonshot Event, Institute for Health Policy, Management and Evaluation, University of Toronto, Canada, http://choir.berkeley.edu/. Accessed November 20, 2014.

[8]   McClellan M, Kent J, Beales S, Cohen SI, Macdonnell M, Thoumi A, Abdulmalik M, Darzi A. Accountable care around the world: A framework to guide reform strategies. *Health Aff (Millwood)*. 2014; 33(9): 1507-1515.

[9]   Behavioural Supports Ontario, Hamilton Niagara Haldimand Brant Local Health Integration Network, BSP Update, June-July, 2014, http://www.hnhblhin.on.ca/ goalsandachievements/integrationpopulationbased/olderadultstheirfamiliesandcaregiver s/supportforfamiliesandcaregivers/BehaviouralSupports.aspx. Accessed December 15, 2014.

[10] National Survey of Accountable Care Organizations, Dartmouth-Berkeley, October 2012 – May 2013. http://choir.berkeley.edu/. Accessed November 20, 2014.

[11] Defining the PCMH. PCMH Resource Center. Agency for Healthcare Research and Quality website. http://pcmh.ahrq.gov/page/defining-pcmh. Accessed November 20, 2014.

[12] Croghan TW, Brown JD. Integrating Mental Health Treatment Into the Patient Centered Medical Home. *AHRQ Publication No. 10-0084-EF*. Rockville, MD: Agency for Healthcare Research and Quality, June 2010.

[13] Behavioral Health Homes for People with Mental Health & Substance Use Conditions: The Core Clinical Features. SAMHSA-HRSA Center for Integrated Health Solutions. Washington, DC, May 2012.

[14] Druss BG, Rohrbaugh RM, Levinson CM, Rosenheck RA. Integrated medical care for patients with serious psychiatric illness: A randomized trial. *Arch Gen Psychiatry* 2001; 58(9): 861-868.

INDEX

Montreal Cognitive Assessment (MoCA), 37
mood stabilizers, xii, 12, 78, 103, 108
multidisciplinary treatment plan, 146

N

National Epidemiological Study on Alcohol and
    Related Conditions (NESARC), 26
neurocognitive disorder, 7, 10, 35, 46, 48, 52, 54,
    101, 131
neuroticism, 15, 16, 17, 18, 20, 54
Nidotherapy, 89, 94, 95, 97, 98
N-methyl-D-aspartate (NMDA), 116
not criminally responsible, 86
not guilty by reason of insanity, 86

O

obesity, 44, 47, 48, 49, 91
Olanzapine, 105, 106
older adults, v, xv, 4, 7, 8, 9, 10, 12, 13, 18, 21, 23,
    26, 28, 29, 34, 37, 41, 43, 44, 45, 46, 47, 48, 52,
    53, 54, 56, 72, 74, 75, 76, 81, 82, 85, 87, 89, 90,
    91, 92, 97, 99, 101, 102, 103, 104, 106, 108, 116,
    131, 132, 134, 135, 138, 143, 146, 152
opioid dependence, 8, 45
opioid pain medications, 44, 45, 48
orthostatic hypotension, xi, 101, 104, 105

P

pain management, 48, 55, 123, 126
Paliperidone, 109
palliative care, 123, 124, 126, 127, 128
paranoid, 18, 19, 83, 84, 92, 94
Patient Protection and Affordable Care Act of 2010,
    148
patient-centered, xvi, 125, 143, 144, 151
Paul Wellstone and Pete Domenici Mental Health
    Parity and Addiction Equality Act of 2008
    (MHPAEA), 148, 149, 150
Personality Assessment Inventory (PAI), 53, 54, 55
Personality Diagnostic Questionnaire, 19, 56, 57
personality disorder, ix, xv, xvi, 3, 4, 5, 6, 8, 9, 10,
    11, 12, 13, 15, 18, 19, 20, 21, 22, 23, 24, 25, 26,
    27, 28, 29, 33, 34, 35, 40, 43, 45, 48, 49, 50, 51,
    52, 54, 56, 57, 61, 65, 68, 69, 71, 78, 79, 80, 81,
    82, 84, 85, 87, 88, 89, 90, 92, 93, 94, 96, 97, 98,
    99, 107, 108, 109, 111, 112, 115, 118, 119, 120,
    124, 128, 131, 132, 133, 134, 135, 136, 137, 138,
    139, 146, 147

personality traits, 6, 8, 10, 15, 16, 18, 21, 22, 50, 53,
    54, 57, 119, 132, 133, 135, 136
pharmacokinetics, 101
phenelzine, 102
Physician Order for Life-Sustaining Treatments, 125
placebo effect, 100, 115, 116
polypharmacy, 101, 143
posttraumatic stress disorder, 4, 10, 13, 43, 44
premature death, 27, 28
protective factors, 72, 75, 76, 78
psychological factors, 24
Psychological Screening Measures, 53
Psychometric Rating Scales, 37
psychostimulants, 106, 116

Q

quality of life, ix, 7, 21, 27, 72, 123, 124, 126, 127,
    131, 136
Quetiapine, 105, 106, 109

R

Reasons for Living Scale – Older Adult Version, 76
repetitive Transcranial Magnetic Stimulation
    (rTMS), 111, 113, 115, 120
Risperidone, 157

S

schema focused therapy, 90
schizoid, 133
self-harm, 9, 10, 24, 25, 34, 36, 38, 44, 45, 47, 52,
    54, 62, 63, 64, 71, 72, 74, 75, 76, 78, 92, 133, 135
self-harming behaviors, 34, 38, 47, 72
self-regulation, 62, 139
sham-controlled trials, 113
somatization, 7
splitting, xvi, 5, 20, 34, 36, 74, 84, 92, 124, 141, 144
Screening Tool in Older Persons for Potentially
    Inappropriate Prescriptions (STOPP), 102
Structured Clinical Interview for DSM Disorders, 53
Substance Abuse and Mental Health Service
    Administration-Health Resources and Services
    Administration (SAMHSA-HRSA), 152, 153
substance use disorder, xv, 4, 43, 44, 45, 48, 49, 100,
    148, 149
suicidal ideation, xi, 10, 13, 36, 37, 67, 72, 74, 75,
    76, 78, 92, 100, 103, 105, 114, 116, 118
suicide, 4, 5, 19, 35, 37, 38, 67, 71, 72, 73, 74, 75,
    76, 78, 79, 80, 91, 92, 101, 118
supportive therapy, 90, 91, 96